Legal Notice

Welcome to Common Sense Labs!

We (Dr. Ken Berry and Kim Howerton) can not and do not attempt to diagnose, treat or cure medical conditions through this book or any discussions arising from this book. Our intention is to give examples and education that can be used as information that you discuss with your doctor - but should never REPLACE the advice of your doctor.

We have written this book as a guide designed to give you general educational information. It has NOT been designed to provide any specific medical advice or diagnoses.
The information provided in this book is not intended to replace the care of a trusted medical practitioner.

Ken Berry, MD and/or Kim Howerton, as authors of this book, shall not be liable to you or anyone else for loss or injury caused in whole or part through decisions made or actions taken, or not taken, due to your interpretation of information provided herein.

Also, please keep in mind that reference ranges shift over time, so there might be discrepancies between what they were at the time of the book publication and when you read it.

Sincerely,
Ken D. Berry, MD and Kim Howerton

....

Common Sense Labs: Blood Labs Demystified
Copyright @2023 Kim Howerton & Ken Berry, MD.

All rights reserved. No part of this book may be reproduced or used in any manner without the permission of the copyright holders.

TABLE OF CONTENTS

1 **Section 1: What Everyone Should Know About Labs**
2 The Problem We Saw
4 The Scope of this Book
5 Basic Terminology
6 Reference Intervals
9 Confounders
11 How to Prep for Your Labs
12 Interpreting Your Labs
14 What to do When Your Doctor Says No
15 ICD-10 Codes

16 **Section 2: Labs to Look at Annually**
17 Common Lab Recommendations are Often Insufficient
20 Annual Labs Details
21 CMP
25 CBC w Diff
28 Lipid Panel
30 Individual Test
37 Metabolic Matters

39 **Section 3: Labs to Check if you are Symptomatic**
40 But What if I am Not Symptom Free
41 Commonly Reported Symptoms
42 Master Hormones & Systems
43 Symptoms & Testing
44 Thyroid
51 Sex Hormones
53 Parathyroid
55 Diagnosis of Exclusion

57 **Section 4: Blood Sugar Monitoring**
59 Glucose Monitoring
60 Targeted Blood Sugar Ranges
62 MAGE
63 Postprandial Blood Sugar

66 **Section 5: Labs Reference Charts - US Units**
67 Annual Labs:
67 CMP
68 CBC w Diff
69 Lipids
69 Urinanalysis
70 Individual Tests
72 Thyroid
73 Sex Hormones

75 **Section 5: Labs Reference Charts - SI Units**
76 Annual Labs
76 CMP
77 CBC w Diff
78 Lipids
78 Urinanalysis
79 Individual Tests
81 Thyroid
82 Sex Hormones

84 **Thank You**
85 **About the Authors**

Section 1:
What Everyone Should Know About Blood Labs

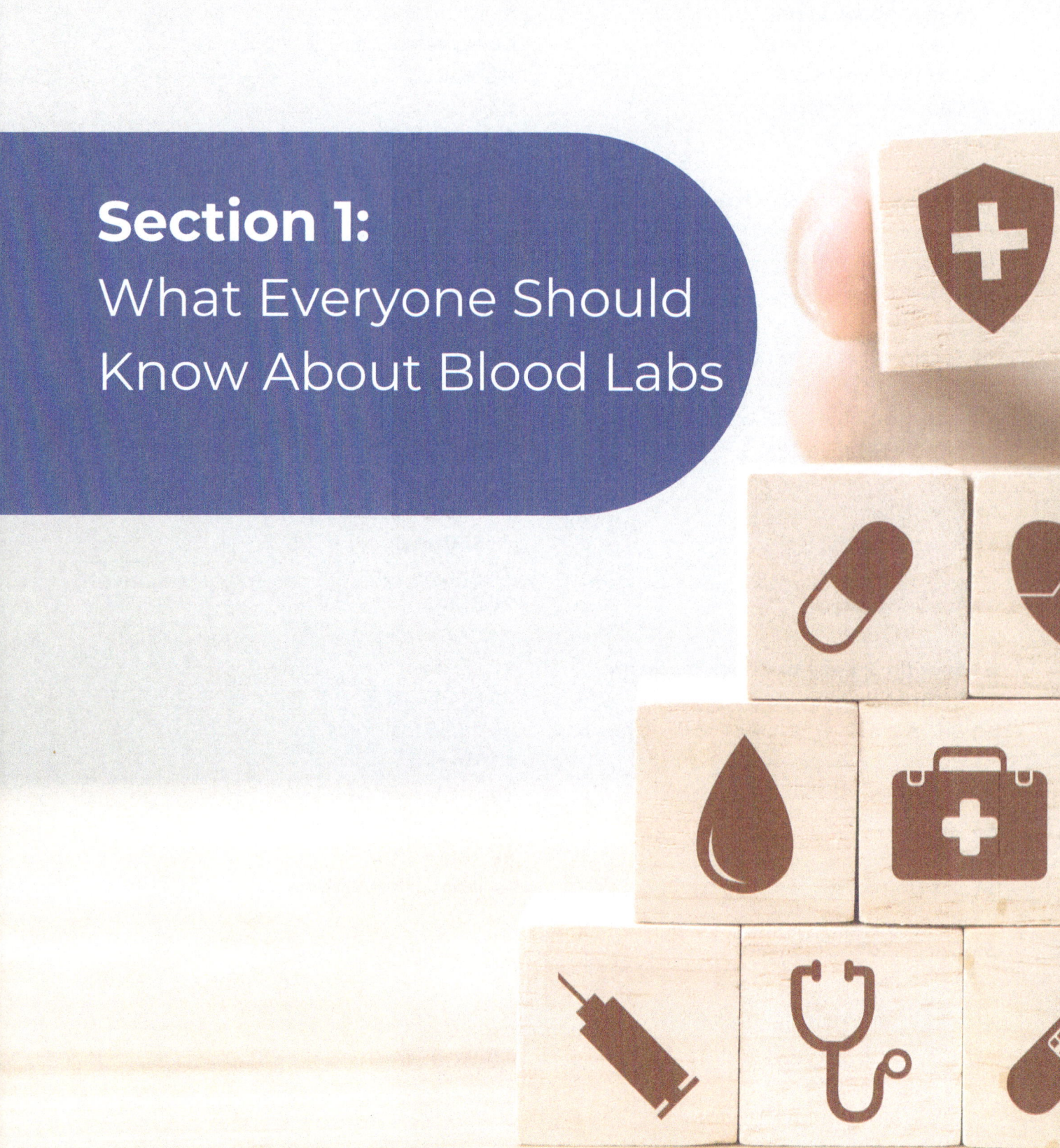

THE PROBLEM WE SAW

Tell me if you've heard this one before...
The doctor send the patient to the phlebotomy lab. A few weeks later, they get a call from a nurse who says, "Your cholesterol is high, so we sent a prescription to the pharmacy."
No further explanation is given. When they ask for clarification, the office tells them the doctor can discuss it with them at the next visit... in 6 months.

Or what about this one?
The receptionist sends an email that says, "Everything on your labs looks fine. The doctor says to try harder to eat right and exercise." But the patient is exhausted no matter how much they sleep, their hair is falling out and they can't seem to get their weight to budge even though they are exercising and eating the way the doctor said to.

Or this one?
A patient tells their doctor they are worried about their diabetes risk and asks for a more comprehensive blood evaluation, but the doctor won't order any more tests because "Your fasting glucose is fine!"

Many of us grew up watching our grandparents (or parents) suffer because they were unwilling or simply unable to question the opinion of their doctor. For years, there was no easy option to become our own health advocate. Our options were limited as most resources were out of reach.

Times have changed. In this modern age, information can be found no farther than the tips of your fingers upon your keyboard. Unfortunately, many blessings bring their own challenges. The Internet is great at information delivery, but this is only part of the process. We all know someone who put their symptoms of runny nose and headache into Dr. Google and determined they have...

CANCER! No- wait... that can't be right, can it?

And here's the rub – information is not enough. Understanding requires context and structure, not just memorizing facts. You can also fall prey to info overload. Unless you understand what things mean, you won't be able to tell the useful from the useless.
This is why it is so critical to have the counsel of a well-informed medical provider – a partner in our health – to really understand the nuance in interpreting our health information.

If anyone is thinking we are arguing for a world without doctors, think again. We love good doctors. What we are arguing for is creating empowered and educated patients working in partnership with their informed and up-to-date doctors.

Dr. B:

For years, I was an ignorant doctor. I mean it, ignorant. I was sure I knew what I knew, and sure those who disagreed with me were idiots. I went to medical school - I studied these things. Surely what I had been taught was right. Right?

"Your cholesterol is high - you need a statin, because high cholesterol will kill you - DUH."

"Your TSH is fine. Your thyroid is fine. Maybe you're tired because you need to lose some weight. DUH."

As we come to expect more from ourselves as active participants in our health journey, we seek to be in partnership with a doctor who will meet us in the spirit of inquiry and experimentation.

Unfortunately, we are aware that not all doctors currently practicing are willing to hold up their end of this bargain – it should be your doctor's role to be your health advocate, not your health roadblock.

There are myriad reasons why patients experience less than optimal care, especially around ordering the right labs. It's rarely because the doctor doesn't care. Most doctors become doctors because they want to help people. Unfortunately, sometimes doctors fall short due to one or more of the following reasons:

- Doctors are often inadequately or inappropriately trained on some labs, "I don't know how to interpret that XYZ lab so I won't order it."
- Many doctors are not up to date on recent developments in lab interpretation since they graduated from Med School many years prior.
- Inappropriately motivated: given motivation by insurance companies to treat in specific ways through billing guidelines.
- Distracted and/or overworked.
- Health Insurance hand slapping – repeatedly being censured by insurance companies for ordering "unnecessary" tests.

We firmly believe in a future of empowered health partnerships, ones in which both lived experience and medical knowledge come together to create optimal health.

Fortunately, the number of plugged-in, forward-thinking doctors is growing. A good doctor will eventually see the light if they are truly committed to improving patients' health.

If your doctor isn't supporting you in the way you need, it might be time to evaluate if your doctor needs education – or if it's time to find a new one that will support you properly.

Dr. B:

But over the years, as my own health declined, and my weight increased, and as I continued to follow and give the "standard" advice that I'd been taught, I realized that something was very wrong.

I became a doctor to help people BE HEALTHIER, and yet following my own advice, I was getting sicker and fatter and just plain old before my time.

I realized I'd become that jaded asshole doctor because I was frustrated. My advice wasn't working, and since my doctor colleagues assured me my advice was sound - so the problem must be my patients' compliance, not my clearly solid advice. But the niggling feeling that this was all wrong wouldn't leave me.

So, I hit my old textbooks, looking for answers. The basis of my medical education was founded on solid biochemistry and physiology - the science. There is a real and true underpinning of science in medical interpretations that are crucial to optimize our health.

What is required, however, is not to simply trust averages, generalities, and ranges without fully investigating the core principles of those tests. Because a lot of what I was saying was, frankly, ridiculous. And I have spent every day of my life since then making up for that by making sure folks know how to actually improve their health.

THE SCOPE OF THIS BOOK

We want regular folks to feel informed and comfortable with their body and medical topics. Since many people have experienced a lot of frustration dealing with medical professionals around the topic of blood testing, we wrote this book for you.

We wanted to solve these kinds of problems, by providing descriptions of common blood tests, what they test for, as well as explaining the results in a user friendly manner. With a more solid understanding, it is our hope that you become more confident and feel like an empowered health partner, not just a passive patient to your healthcare provider.

Think of blood lab interpretation as layers.
In the first layer, you have the tests that confirm a good health foundation. This Level 1 grouping of tests covers basic health markers that should be checked regularly to confirm that you continue to maintain a baseline of foundational good health. This will be covered in section 2, starting on page 16.

A second layer would touch on deeper topics, such as testing someone might consider when complaining of some of the more common symptoms that Dr. Berry would see in the clinic, which we discuss in section 3. These tests include concerns such as thyroid dysregulation and sex hormone abnormalities.

There are many more layers that we do not approach in this book. Interpreting complex labs requires much more nuance and multi-factor analysis, and we felt it was way beyond the scope of what should be tackled in this book.

By getting clear on the basics, we hope that what we give you in this book provides a rock-solid foundation to stand on if you ever need to delve deeper into more complex health topics with your medical provider.

Kim:

My story is a little different than Dr. Berry's, not the story of a doctor, but a patient. I had my first surgery at 5, was diagnosed with depression at 9, PCOS at 15, and spent most of my young(ish) life suffering from undiagnosed hypothyroidism. Gastritis by 17, followed by ongoing irritable bowel syndrome. Not to mention my ever-worsening eating disorder and growing weight issues.

It turns out that undiagnosed hypothyroidism was a lynchpin, and it took me two decades to get properly diagnosed. When it finally was, the world shifted for me. Those of you who live with chronic illness probably understand the difference between a good day and a bad day, and when I was undiagnosed, it was almost always a bad day.

The one-two punch of overhauling what I ate and properly balancing my thyroid levels changed my world. I would not have been able to experience this without doing a deep dive into the labs that actually matter and partnering with a doctor who helped me get properly medicated.

As of the writing of this book, I'm down over 100 pounds and experiencing clarity and energy that I never imagined I could feel in my sicker days.

I want all of you reading this to be TRULY empowered on your health journey.

BASIC TERMINOLOGY

Starting with the basics means making sure that we are clear on terms. Some of you already may be familiar with these terms, but a large part of the problem people encounter with medical professionals is they use a lot of unfamiliar words and phases. This use of jargon can often create a gap between those "in the know" and the general public. Throughout this book we will do our best to cut through the jargon and discuss concepts using clear terms and explanations.

> Jargon: "Special words or expressions that are used by a particular profession or group and are difficult for others to understand."
> *Oxford Languages*

Common Sense Labs Terms

Biomarker or Marker: An isolated indicator used to identify, predict or characterize health status. This could refer to a marker within a blood test, but can also refer to other health testing, for example: blood pressure is considered a biomarker.

Blood Draw: The act of getting blood taken (drawn) from the body.

Blood Work: Another way to refer to the examination of a blood test.

Lab: Short for Laboratory. A location equipped with equipment to run testing and analysis.

Labs: While it could be the plural of the above definition of Lab, it is more often used to refer to Lab tests or Lab Test results. As many terms are shortened to the word "Labs," you'll need to look at the context to understand specifically what is being referred to. Examples: "Have you done your Labs?" "What did your Labs say?"

Lab Sample: Body fluid (such as a blood or urine) or tissue collected for the purpose of testing. Blood samples can be taken from veins (venous) from an artery (arterial) or from a finger tip, or in the case of an infant the heel (capillary). Most blood tests are run from venous samples.

Lab Test: A procedure run in a lab by a health care professional in which a lab sample is extracted for the purpose of testing and a specific test is run on that sample.

Phlebotomy: The act of puncturing a vein to draw blood. A person who does this by trade is called a phlebotomist.

Serum: A blood sample with specific clotting factors removed. Many rests are run specifically on serum samples. A lab will use a centrifuge (a mechanical device) to separate the parts of the blood blood to create a serum sample.

Enzyme: Proteins that act as catalysts within the body, to start, speed, slow or stop biological processes.

Proxy: A stand-in. In the case of blood tests, usually means a marker that is more easily measured used to estimate a related marker.

WHAT ARE REFERENCE INTERVALS?

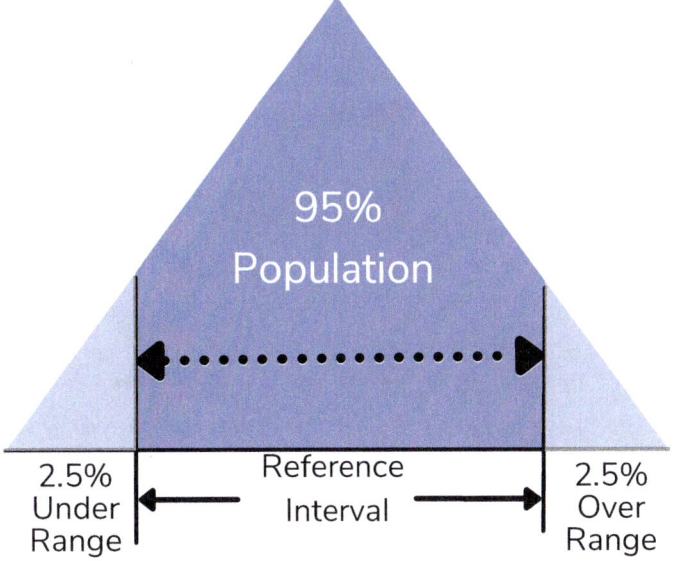

We assume most of you have, at some time, had blood work done. Your doctor has given you paperwork, you went to a lab and had blood drawn, and the doctor's office called with the results. Some of you might even have been sent the results showing you what is in and out of "range."

First, some terminology:
On lab paperwork you'll often see the term "reference interval." Your test results will be classified as within or outside this range. A reference interval might also be called a reference range or standard range. A reference interval is determined by taking the lab results for a population and then putting them on a mathematical curve. As you see in the image above, this curve excludes the bottom and top 2.5% - which means that the reference interval reflects the range of results of 95% of the population. This range of values is then considered "normal" within a population - on some lab results they even go as far as using the word "normal" when defining reference ranges, although we argue it would be better to call it common, rather than use the term "normal."

Reference range data is drawn from a group of people that have taken a specific test. While an effort is generally made to remove the data of those with known illnesses, that is not always possible. This is due to the reality that the general population is rife with undiagnosed medical issues. Therefore, the reference range will include some of the population that probably should have been excluded due to illness. Many tests also have specific ranges for subsets like age, ethnicity, and/or sex.

There are also some reasons you might see differences in reference ranges. Ranges may often vary slightly between lab companies. You'll also sometimes find some regional differences in quoted ranges. And of course, as we discuss in the section on Historical Ranges, these reference intervals vary over time as population level health shifts.

Not all ranges are determined by calculating the 95% reference interval, some are determined by "consensus." Meaning a medical governing body has set the range, so it's not exclusively based on population statistics.
Blood Glucose and Lipid recommendations are examples of this type.

REFERENCE RANGE PROBLEMS

You may have gotten bloodwork results presented in chart form as you see here.

Most folks would assume that if they got this result of 43 on a GGT lab result, it would be reasonable to interpret that to mean their level was good. After all, it's in range!

GGT (gamma-glutamyl transferase) is a key liver marker, which we will describe in more detail in section 2. This chart depicts that any number between 3-55 is considered "in range" at this lab. Which might lead a person to believe if their GGT was anywhere between 3 and 55, they are equally healthy. After all, there's no degree of greenness showing here, it's black and white... err green and red. There's no super-green and sorta-green.

However, this "everything in the range is good" assumption is far from reality. In practice, having a high GGT is known to be an indicator of either current or likely future liver damage. Many functional medicine doctors aren't happy seeing GGT levels over 30. So why does this report consider anything up to 55 "normal"? **The answer is the 95% curve... the reference range.**

Reference ranges are a reflection of the health within a society.
Less than 12% of the US population qualifies as metabolically healthy, and yet, for the majority of that unhealthy 88%, this fact would not disqualify them from being included in the reference ranges. It would only be when their condition had advanced to clearly diseased that they might be excluded... maybe.

And what is the cost we pay as patients?

We end up being told that "You're fine! All your blood work came back normal!" when we feel anything but fine.
Understanding how these ranges were set can help us have better discussions with our doctors, and hopefully receive useful medical intervention when needed.

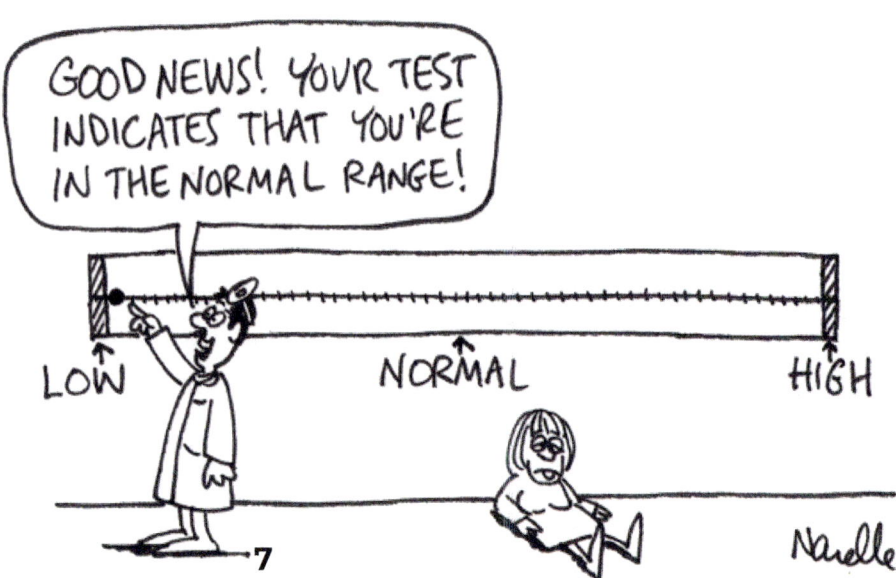

LAB RANGES SHIFT OVER TIME

What? Reference intervals change? Well, if you think about it, it makes sense. Most folks have never considered that ranges will change as the health of the population shifts,

To illustrate the issue with historical ranges, we will start with an example - **Testosterone!**

What is testosterone? It is a sex hormone found in both men and women, though in much higher amounts in men. When looking at annual averages, numbers for men have been declining at about a rate of 1% per year.

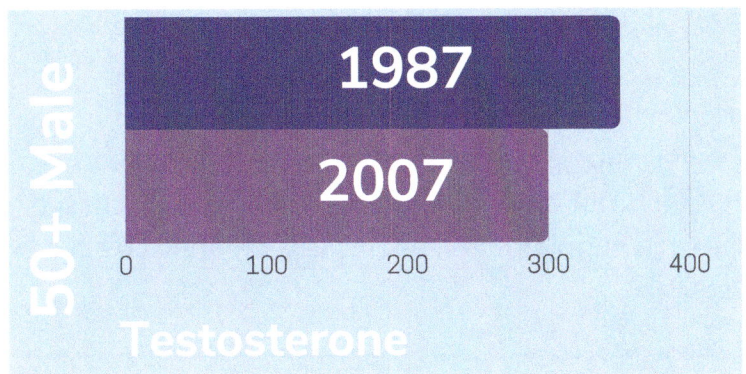

Average Testosterone levels of a 60-year-old man in 1987 vs 2007.

(Journal of Clinical Endocrinology and Metabolism, 2007)

Reference ranges dropping in concert - not because men are healthier with lower testosterone, but because "Low T" is becoming the new normal.

The reference range was not lowered because the medical establishment had come to the realization that lower Testosterone is better. As the average Testosterone level in the population has declined, the reference range has dropped to reflect that. This is true of countless test ranges.

Ultimately, it's clear that in a population suffering from ever-declining health, population-based reference ranges are not a good yardstick for optimal health.

While some reference ranges mirror the optimal range, you can't assume that to be true for the reference range for each test. In evaluating whether your doctor will optimize your health, be sure to discuss with your doctor what they consider to be optimal with respect to reference ranges for each of your tests.

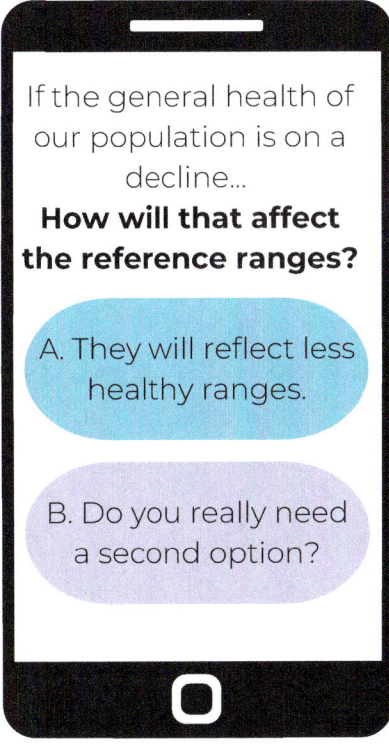

If the general health of our population is on a decline...
How will that affect the reference ranges?

A. They will reflect less healthy ranges.

B. Do you really need a second option?

CONFOUNDERS

WHAT IS A CONFOUNDER?

There are a variety of substances and actions that can obscure or change your test results, causing the results to be incorrect or misleading. These are considered confounders. The top confounders for blood tests are medications and supplements, but there can also be significant effects from your dietary or hydration patterns. In general, it's considered a confounder when it can affect the outcome of the test, potentially leading to erroneous interpretations, but not causing actual health issues.

Here are some often overlooked confounders in blood lab testing:

BIOTIN: Biotin interferes with several blood tests, including SHBG, thyroid tests, progesterone tests, B-12, and others. All biotin supplementation should be discontinued 3-5 days before any testing, or if discontinuation is not advised, the topic should be discussed with your doctor. There are several multivitamin supplements that include biotin, so be sure to review your supplements' ingredient lists.

CREATINE: Can be increased with supplemental creatine or from a diet very high in red meat. This can artificially elevate Creatinine and eGFR results. Discuss with your doctor if they become concerned with a higher-than-expected creatinine level. Increased Creatinine levels do not always reflect poor kidney function. Other markers can be looked at instead to assess kidney function, such as CystatinC, in the case of a diet high in protein and/or creatinine.

IRON: If you are looking at Ferritin or Iron levels, the general advice is to discontinue the use of any iron supplements for 5 days before the test. If the test is ordered by your doctor, make sure they agree with this and aren't expecting you to be on your normal dose at the time of testing.

ILLNESS & EXERTION: If you've been ill or had an injury or infection before testing, this could cause your inflammation markers to be extremely elevated. Additionally, hard exercise too close to the day of the test could have a similar effect.

DEHYDRATION: Aside from making the blood draw itself difficult, tests are based on blood concentration, which means if you are dehydrated, levels can look artificially high due to low blood volume. Make sure in the days leading up to, and the day of the draw, you are properly hydrated.

CONFOUNDERS

HOW CAN DIETARY PATTERNS AFFECT RESULTS?

It shouldn't come as a surprise to readers who are familiar with the authors that we think that a proper diet is a central part of a healthy life, with a definite preference for what some would call a low-carbohydrate diet. Though this book is meant to be useful regardless of diet type, we felt it important to point out a few common things we see when people improve their eating habits.

As we discussed on previous pages, the reference range is based on the average American, and in our opinion, the average American is not eating a healthy diet. In many cases, an improved diet will improve blood markers. However, there are some ways of eating that can make a blood marker misleading or confusing when we use folks on a SAD diet (Standard American Diet) as the norm. Sometimes following what we consider a healthier eating pattern can influence blood markers in a way that puts them out of range when the range is based on SAD eating patterns.

Most notably, as the average American (especially women) eats too little protein, and a higher protein diet can change BUN (Blood Urea Nitrogen) or Creatinine in ways that can erroneously cause alarm when reviewing blood labs. Because these labs do not distinguish between protein in serum caused by kidney dysfunction (which is very bad) and higher protein due to eating more protein (which is not bad), it's good to know this.

In terms of low-carb diets, there are some markers that will still be within the reference range, but can trend lower on the range, such as blood sugar, insulin and c-peptide. Additionally, some have reported their T3 (a thyroid marker) is slightly lower than they'd see on a high carb diet, but remain asymptomatic (having no symptoms) of thyroid dysfunction.

Additionally, as you might already know, for some folks, generally known as 'hyper-responders' - LDL (low density lipoproteins, which will be discussed in section 2) can be significantly raised for some following a low-carb diet. While this may or may not be something that concerns you, being aware of the tendencies can help you best evaluate your health status.

In no way are we suggesting ignoring these levels if they come back out of range. We simply raise the topic to make sure you are informed that some of your labs might look slightly different based on your food choices. If you have concerns, do not hesitate to discuss your concerns with your doctor about the ways that your food or hydration level may have affected the testing. If a test comes back unexpectedly out of range, ask them if retesting is a good idea.

HOW TO PREP FOR YOUR LABS:
What to Expect

Water only 12-14 hours prior to test

Common Sense Labs Prep

As mentioned in Confounders, you want to be properly hydrated when going in for your blood draw. Ask your medical provider if you need guidance in terms of proper hydration.

Some labs need to be run "fasted" and some do not. What does fasted mean?

In this case, fasting means not eating or drinking anything except water. We recommend that you do not eat or drink anything except water and possibly salt (this includes no coffee!) in the 12-14 hours before your test. Because it's easy to get confused about whether tests need to be fasted or not, we actually advise you to assume all tests should be done fasted, unless you are specifically testing a response to eating.

In this SAD eating world where most folks seem to feel the need to eat every 3 hours, fasting for blood work has begun to be thought of as torturous. Because of this, some doctors have started saying it doesn't matter if you are fasted, but we know of many situations in which a patient was prescribed unnecessary medications based on their non-fasted numbers. There can be a huge downside to allowing some tests to be done when not fasted, especially if you eat a low-carb diet, non-fasted numbers can be inordinately out of range on these diets, whereas fasted numbers show a more accurate picture.

When we say 12-14 hours, that is no less than 12, but no more than 14. Even if you are someone who usually has a longer fasting window, now is not the time to do so. This is because some tests look increasingly out of range after longer fasting windows (LDL is one example). If you have a 9am test, you want to be finished with dinner no earlier than 7pm, and no later than 9pm.

If you regularly work out in the mornings, we'd suggest skipping your workout on the day of the draw. As mentioned in **Confounders**, a workout, especially a hard one, can artificially elevate some lab results. For standard workouts, just skipping that day is all that needs to be altered. If you've done any major exercise, such as participating in a marathon, give it a few days before doing blood work to allow inflammatory markers to return to normal.

Additionally, discuss with your doctor how they want you to handle taking or not taking any medications the morning of the blood draw, as this can affect how they interpret results regarding related markers.

INTERPRETING YOUR LABS

LAB RANGES
Once your labs come in, your doctor will look at your test results and compare them to the known reference ranges. There are several reasons why labs are delineated in ranges rather than aiming for a specific target number. First, there is variability person to person, some might naturally run a little higher, some a little lower on any given marker. Even within one individual, there will be some day to day variation, as the human body is a living and changing entity. Daily shifts in nutrition, hydration, sleep and many other factors will cause subtle, or sometimes not so subtle, shifts in blood chemistry. This means that we aim to be within a range, not a singular number. This is one reason that it's important to get regular bloodwork, so you'll be able to recognize it if you start to see a significant departure from what is normal for you.

We believe that many standard ranges are too widely set, which makes using the optimal range especially important. In this book, we base our discussions on Dr. Berry's optimal ranges. This does not mean that your doctor's ranges are wrong if they are not identical. However, a good doctor should have questioned the reference ranges and have developed their own preference in what they hope to see, not just automatic acceptance of the common ranges. You'll find in our reference charts in sections 5 & 6, sometimes the standard reference interval is appropriate for evaluating your lab work, but often there's a tighter range we believe people should aim for.

DIRECT VS. ESTIMATED RESULTS
There are two methods of determining test results: direct and estimated. Direct measures the specific quantity of a substance within the lab sample. Estimated results do not test that marker directly, but instead use a calculation to determine the estimated value based on a surrogate marker instead. This is sometimes also referred to as indirect testing or a calculated result. We bring this to your attention as we find that while estimated results are often fine, in some cases a calculated result can return less accurate information as they depend on more assumptions.

For example, most blood work includes a GFR, which is a glomerular filtration rate. This marker is a measure of how well your kidneys are filtering. Almost always, what is reported is an eGFR - the e indicating estimated. While a dGFR (direct glomerular filtration rate) can be run, it is a very complicated process and impractical in most circumstances. The problem that can arise with the estimated form is that calculation is based on creatinine levels. Creatinine is a waste product from the normal breakdown of muscle tissue as well as the digestion of dietary protein. As we mentioned in Confounders, Creatinine levels can also be affected by the ingestion of some supplements as well as how much muscle mass a person has.

INTERPRETING YOUR LABS

The Creatinine level that was used to estimate the GFR is a direct measure test. It measures how much creatinine is in your blood. But it doesn't explain why it's high or low. For that, your doctor (and you) will need to evaluate the level based on an understanding of your specific circumstances. This is an example of why you must look at blood results within the proper context. Blood work simply tells us what is in the blood - not why it is there. Here are a few different reasons your Creatinine could be high:
1. Your kidneys are impaired.
2. You lift weights a lot and have a lot of muscle mass.
3. You eat a lot of meat.
4. You take supplemental Creatine.

As you can see, an eGFR could return a result suggesting that there might be a problem with your kidneys, when it's actually just an artifact of a higher protein diet. Conversely to the alarm this might raise, this higher protein intake may actually lead to healthier kidneys. It's important to know that any estimated value can be inaccurate depending on circumstance. The results can still be potentially useful, but take them with a grain of salt.

You also might not know which markers on your labs are estimated vs. directly measured. Not all will be listed with an **e** added. Other common examples of estimated results are A1C (sometimes called eAG - estimated average glucose because it's used to estimate your average glucose), and some lipids such as an LDL-C, where the C stands for calculated.

When your doctor is looking at your labs, they are generally looking for anything that stands out as unexpected or out of range. They will also pay attention to values that seem discordant, that is they don't match up with their examination or your other blood results. They might then follow-up to diagnose or eliminate concerns. Doctors are taught, "when you hear hoofbeats, expect horses, not zebras," a phrase that means, don't go for the exotic diagnosis when a common one is much more likely. However, if a common diagnosis is ruled out, and the issue persists, make sure your doctor keeps looking.

In this book, we mainly discuss basic labs that a doctor should run if you do not have any significant health complaints. While it generally goes beyond what we can do here in this book to work with specific problems, we will talk about some common patterns that present themselves in the clinic when someone is feeling less than optimal. You'll find that discussion in section 3.

Common Sense Labs wants you to know:
Lab Tests aren't always perfectly accurate. Though they are more accurate than most at-home test kits, lab tests still have accepted ranges of accuracy. Also, while not common, there can be lab errors... so if you ever feel like one of your lab results seems wrong, ask to retest.

WHAT TO DO WHEN YOUR DOCTOR SAYS NO

While reading this book, you may find that there are tests you desire that your doctor doesn't support. It's unfortunately common to hear from people that their doctor is resistant to ordering them the labs that they ask to be included. If this is the case with you, it's important to understand why your doctor is resistant so that you can counter their concern properly.

It's common a doctor won't want to order a test because they are unfamiliar with it. They worry they won't know how to interpret the data. However, don't let that stop you, this is an opportunity for both you and your doctor to gain more insight into your health. Ask them if they are open to learning more about a marker you think could be useful to include in your tests.

Or maybe your doctor thinks that your insurance won't pay for certain tests because they don't know how to code them. On the following page we've listed some ICD-10 (International Classification of Disease - 10th edition) codes. These are reference numbers a doctor can submit to insurance to increase the likelihood of getting tests reimbursed. Feel free to share this book with your doctor. Or perhaps it's a test they don't believe will be approved, even if properly coded. If you run into this road block, and are willing to pay cash for the cost of the test, you can tell your doctor you are fine paying directly. Be sure to ask your doctor about the cost of the test in advance.

Doctors are human, but like all humans, can always improve. Requiring your doctor to be perfect is unrealistic. However, your doctor has to be willing to be a partner in answering your questions, concerns and needs. Ultimately, just like in any relationship, you need to consider if there is clear communication, and is this worth the investment, time and energy?

If a doctor refuses a test which you feel you need, tell your doctor to note in your chart their refusal to order the test. Say to your doctor, "I'm worried about my health and feel strongly that the results of this test could be important to me. If you refuse to order this test, please write that you refused this request in my permanent medical record and print me a copy of your refusal." Do not leave the office without the print out. Many health care providers will be hesitant to put their refusal in writing and will hopefully, if reluctantly, order the test for you. Of course, having to take this hard-line approach is likely a signal that your doctor is not the health partner for which you were hoping.

Never forget, this is your one life to live. If your doctor will not work with you - find a new one who is open to being a great partner.

As a last resort, be aware in most US States, individuals can order blood tests directly from testing service companies for fairly reasonable prices. See our resource page for more info: https://commonsenselabslinks.com

Common Sense Insurance Codes: ICD-10

Please note: ICD Codes are standardized numbers used Internationally. These are the codes your doctor would submit for insurance reimbursement. This is a partial list, selected to give you the specific codes Dr. Berry believes are most relevant to this book.

ICD-10 CODES	SYMPTOMS
R53.8	Fatigue
R07.9	Chest Pain
R73.9	Hyperglycemia
E16.2	Hypoglycemia
E88.81	Metabolic Syndrome
R63.5	Abnormal Weight Gain
R63.4	Abnormal Weight Loss
R03.0	Elevated Blood Pressure without Dx
E06.3	Autoimmune Thyroiditis
R68.82	Decreased Libido
E28.310	Menopause Symptoms
E29.1	Hypogonadism
G44.59	Headache
K76.0	Fatty Liver
R10.10	Upper Abdominal Pain
E04.9	Goiter
L30.9	Dermatitis, unspec
R06.02	Shortness of Breath
G31.84	Memory Loss
R45.84	Anhedonia

SECTION 2:
COMMON SENSE LABS TO LOOK AT ANNUALLY

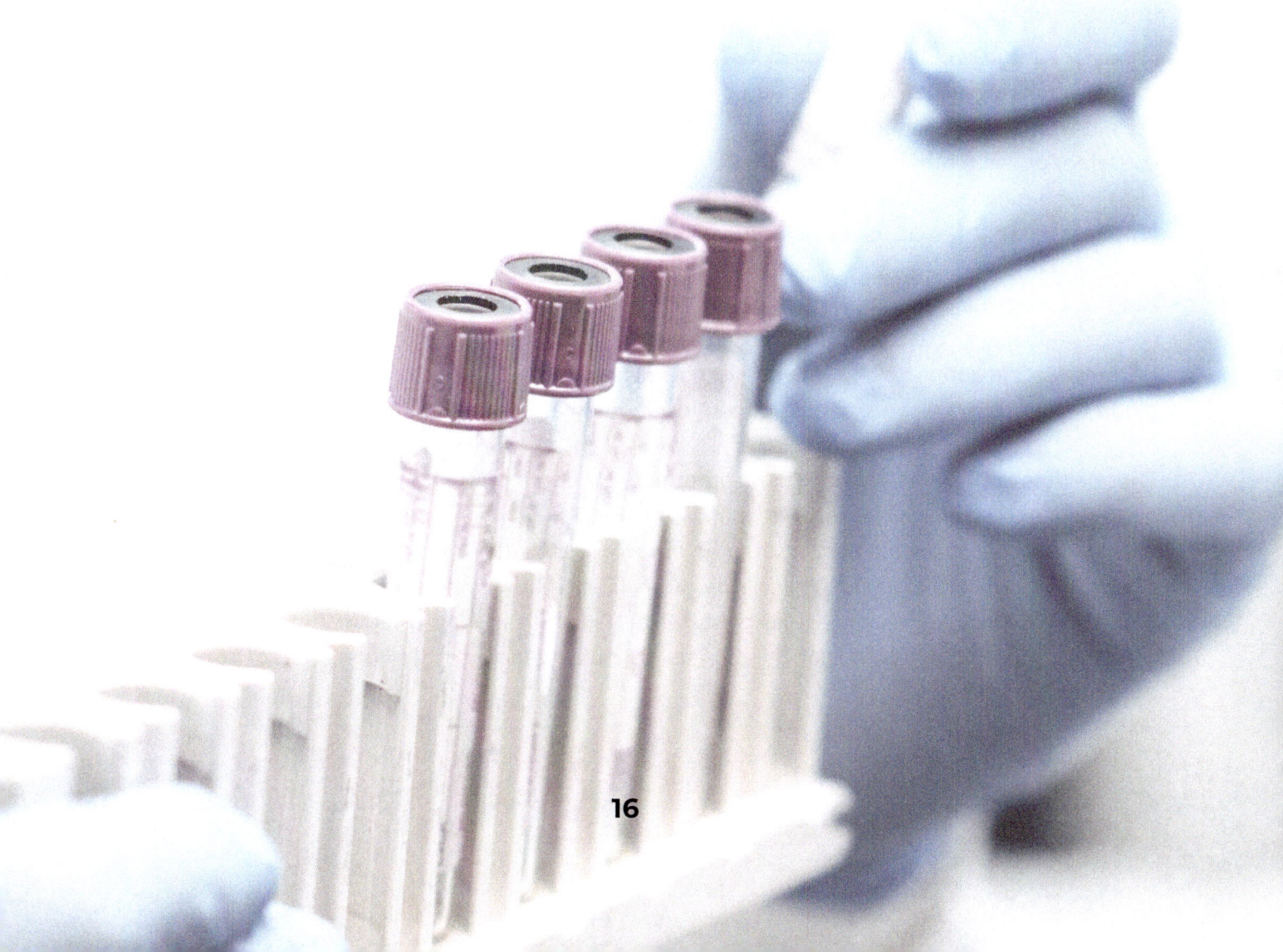

COMMON LAB RECOMMENDATIONS ARE OFTEN INSUFFICIENT

I think we can all agree that a yearly snapshot of our health via blood labs is a great idea. As patients and consumers, we often have no idea what that effective annual snapshot should include.

The list of tests most doctors include in their Annual Labs is frankly inadequate.
In mainstream medicine, an annual order usually looks like this:

- BMP (basic metabolic panel)
- CBC (complete blood count)
- Basic Lipids
- Urinalysis

This is considered comprehensive by most, and in fact, some doctors order even less than this!

But is this really all you need? We don't think so.

Here's the huge problem with checking too few tests: If a doctor is planning to use these labs as the #1 source of objective information on a patient's health, they need to make sure that all the main bases of health are covered. Any given lab in isolation without some supporting confirmation from other labs can result in very inaccurate interpretations of the numbers. In the case that a given lab marker comes back significantly out of range, a good doctor will order a repeat test to confirm it, as it's not impossible there was a lab error.

But think for a minute - does the reverse ever happen? That a doctor looks at an in-range number and says, "Let's confirm that wasn't a lab error." No, that doesn't happen unless there is evidence to the contrary. This is what you get when you are really comprehensive about your blood work - you get some degree of confirmation on all the tests in tandem.

That being said, we will also mention something we find in growing frequency in some alternative medicine circles - over-testing. Wait, didn't you just warn of under-testing? Yep. This is why it is so important to be educated on what labs to get. Many (not all) mainstream practitioners will under-test.. While many (not all) alternative medical practitioners will over-test. There's a goldilocks zone- the right tests to be useful and informative, but not throwing a lengthy and potentially confusing list of tests at you as a means to sell you a ton of supplements that you don't need.

WHY YOU NEED A CMP NOT JUST A BMP

CMP - Comprehensive Metabolic Panel: A CMP is a panel of tests that look at elements of metabolism, kidney and liver health, and basic electrolyte balance.
Many doctors will order a Basic Metabolic Panel (BMP) instead of a Comprehensive one. What's the difference? In basic terms:

BMP is 8 tests whereas **CMP is 14 tests**

What does the Basic miss? Beyond the fact that 14 is more than 8, the reason you should care about that is the BMP excludes two essential markers of Liver health - ALT (alanine transaminase) and AST (aspartate aminotransferase).

Why are ALT and AST so essential? Years ago, the only times we tended to see people with Fatty Liver Disease was when overuse of alcohol or medication was involved. However, in more recent years we've seen an enormous uptick in the diagnosed cases of Non-Alcoholic Fatty Liver Disease (NAFLD). In fact, some have suggested we actually should use the term: MAFLD - *Metabolic Associated* Fatty Liver Disease, because the vast majority of cases are metabolic in nature.

Over 25% of the population has been diagnosed with Fatty Liver Disease, and that's a low estimate, as it's a significantly under-diagnosed disorder. One reason for its under-diagnosis is that most doctors aren't looking for signs in their blood panels, because they order a BMP, not a CMP. We find it incredibly scary that as this condition becomes more common, many doctors are suggesting that fatty liver is really no big deal, because they've grown so accustomed to seeing it. But as we know, in a sick society common doesn't mean healthy.

If left unchecked, Fatty Liver Disease can progress to NASH - Non-Alcoholic SteatoHepatitis - a serious liver condition that will lead to liver failure. Since MAFLD rarely results in obvious symptoms, one needs to be proactively looking for it. And since MAFLD is easily reversible, but NASH is not, early detection matters.

JORDAN'S STORY

Jordan was a model patient, never missing his annual checkup. Then one year at his check-up, he mentioned he has a bit of stomach upset, not to mention a growing gut. His doctor advised him to try to eat better. More whole grains and less bacon, to walk more, and try to lose a few pounds, suggesting that he was suffering from "middle-age spread" as so many men of his age do. Year after year, Jordan went back, hearing the same advice, doing his best to comply – switching his bacon and eggs to whole-wheat toast and oatmeal.

Several years down the line, his doctor was shocked at the change in his appearance. Jordan looked run down and his complexion was tinged with yellow. Concerned, the doctor ordered a liver ultrasound and found Jordan had cirrhosis of the liver – a life-threatening liver condition.

After some research, Jordan realized that years back, those early days of a bit of belly pain and gut distention, that he thought was just some weight gain, were actually very early signs of MAFLD – Metabolic Associated Fatty Liver Disease. This then progressed unchecked to NASH - Non-Alcoholic SteatoHepatitis which then eventually became cirrhosis as the damage continued.

If the doctor had been checking a CMP (complete metabolic panel) and not just a BMP (basic metabolic panel) and had added a GGT to his annual tests, his doctor would have known what was happening under the surface with plenty of time to correct the situation. But now that it had progressed so long and far, Jordan was facing possible liver failure and a need for a liver transplant.

Jordan's doctor was old school, trained when the common cause of Fatty Liver Disease was overuse of alcohol. And since Jordan didn't drink to excess, his doctor didn't even consider that might be an issue.

MAFLD rarely results in symptoms, which makes it crucial to address before it progresses to NASH, which means we need to be actively looking for it.

When ALT and AST are even slightly elevated, it's an indication to look closer at the function of the liver and take active steps to alter the trajectory of liver health. Then we cross-reference that with the results of the GGT, which complements the look into liver function. These conditions can be reversed or prevented with the proper interventions, but unfortunately, because Jordan's doctor never checked, the condition was discovered too late. Jordan is now on the list for a liver transplant.

COMMON SENSE LABS: ANNUAL RECOMMENDATIONS

Up to this point, we've pointed out that the majority of doctors may not be recommending all the right labs for you.

By now, you are likely asking, "So what are the right labs for me?!"

Here is the list of Labs we recommend for everyone over the age of 30 to have checked annually. This "Annual List" is the baseline health check we recommend for everyone to keep an eye on.

In this section we'll go over the annual tests and explain in detail what you need to know to be a well educated patient.

Some of these tests are called Panels. Panels are pre-arranged groups of related tests, as compared to individual tests, which are single labs that can be tested one by one. You'll find a combination of both panels and individual tests on our list.

The first panel we discuss is a CMP - Comprehensive Metabolic Panel, which reports the blood levels of proteins, electrolytes and glucose levels. These tests reflect the health of your liver, kidneys, bones, muscles, nerves, and cell function.

Common Sense Annual Labs List

A1C (related to glucose)
B-12 (vitamin)
Copper (mineral)
CBC w/ Diff (blood cell health)
CMP (metabolite panel)
C-Peptide (related to insulin)
D-25 (vitamin)
DHEA-S (sex hormone)
ESR (related to inflammation)
Fasting Insulin (baseline insulin)
Ferritin (related to iron)
GGT (liver marker)
Homocysteine (amino acid)
hsCRP (related to Inflammation)
Iron (mineral)
Lipid Panel (cholesterol)
Magnesium (electrolyte)
Phosphorous (electrolyte)
TSH (thyroid stimulating hormone)
Uric Acid (inflammatory marker)
Vitamin C (vitamin)
Zinc (mineral)
Urinalysis (related to kidney function)

TESTS WITHIN THE CMP: WHAT THEY MEASURE

Albumin	A liver protein that helps maintain fluid balance in your bloodstream. It is also imperative in vitamin, hormone, and enzyme transport. Out-of-range numbers can indicate kidney or liver disfunction or malnutrition.
Alkaline Phosphatase	Sometimes shortened to ALP, an enzyme used by the body in protein breakdown. Out-of-range numbers can point to dysfunction in one of several organs, most frequently the kidney, liver, bone, gallbladder or intestines.
ALT	(Alanine transaminase) An enzyme made primarily by the liver. While a small amount is found outside the liver, if high quantities are found in the bloodstream this indicates some degree of liver dysfunction.
AST	(Aspartate aminotransferase) An enzyme primarily made in the liver, though also made in small amounts by other organs. Similarly to ALT, if high quantities are in your blood, there is most likely liver impairment of some kind.
Bilirubin	Part of red blood cell breakdown, processed by the liver and then excreted. High levels either mean an issue with red blood cells, such as in sickle cell anemia, or an issue with liver filtration which can indicate liver or bile duct problems.
BUN	(Blood Urea Nitrogen) Another byproduct of kidney function that shows how well your kidneys are working, frequently affected by hydration status. Often evaluated in conjunction with Creatinine. Certain dietary patterns, especially increased protein diets, can impact levels. .
Calcium	An electrolyte. Most people already know it's essential for bone health, but may not know it plays important roles in blood clotting and cell function as well as managing heart rhythm, signaling nerves and regulating muscle contractions. The amount in blood is tightly controlled, and being off, even by a small amount, can indicate health problems.

TESTS WITHIN THE CMP: WHAT THEY MEASURE

Carbon Dioxide	An electrolyte. A waste product related to respiration, blood oxygenation and blood alkilinity. Out-of-range levels can indicate a dysfunction in the kidney or lung.
Chloride	An electrolyte. Tightly aligned with blood sodium levels. Can indicate proper fluid balance, as well as possibly point to some potential syndromes or diseases, though dehydration must be ruled out as that is far more common a cause of being out of range.
Creatinine	An indicator of proper kidney function. It's often viewed in parallel with BUN (Blood Urea Nitrogen) to give a more well-rounded picture. It can be a less useful marker on a high protein diet.
Globulin	There are actually four types of globulins in blood, which are indicated in blood clotting, immune function, and liver function.
Glucose	Also known as Blood Sugar. Varies throughout the day, and changes based on what you've recently eaten. The body very tightly controls levels of glucose in the blood, as being too far out-of-range is extremely dangerous. Consistently high Glucose is an indicator of Diabetes.
pH	This common abbreviation means potential of Hydrogen, as Hydrogen levels determine acidity. Some Labs, but not all, will include a venous pH. This is not your actual blood pH and very seldom returns any useful data.
Potassium	An electrolyte. Essential to muscle health, most critically the heart muscle. It is crucial for electrical signaling to the heart and nervous system. Though all electrolytes interact with each other, Potassium is especially sensitive to Sodium levels, and healthy Potassium levels require a balance with Sodium

TESTS WITHIN THE CMP: WHAT THEY MEASURE

Protein	Total Protein measures the globulin and albumin in your blood. These proteins are essential for cell structure. This test can point to possible liver or kidney problem as well as protein malnutrition.
Sodium	An electrolyte. Crucial for cell fluid balance and proper nerve and electrical signaling. In the absence of extreme circumstances, the body is excellent at maintaining Sodium balance. An imbalance suggests a need for immediate Sodium correction, or if chronically off, might point to a possible kidney issue as the kidneys are crucial for maintaining sodium balance in the blood.

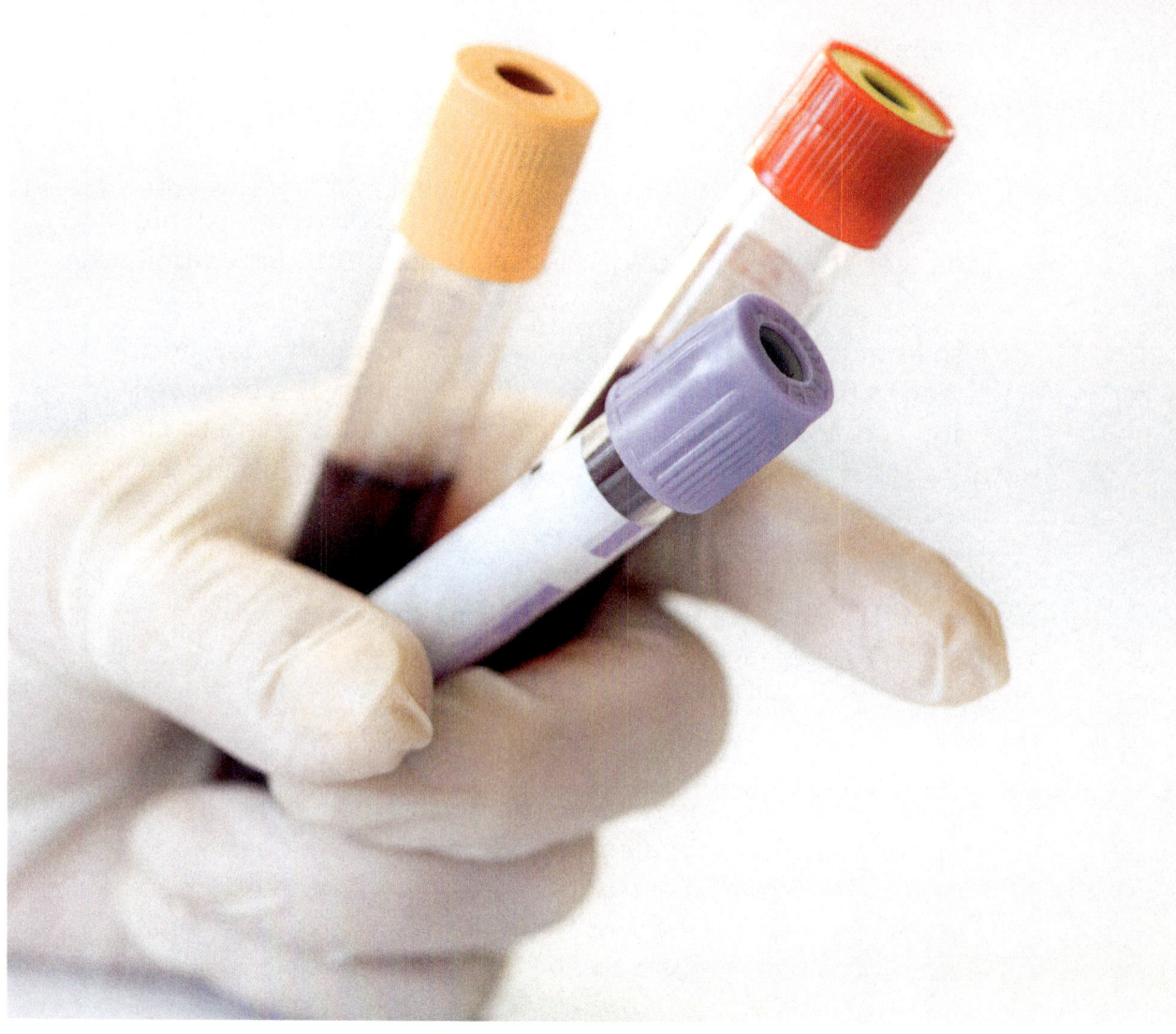

HOW ELECTROLYTE BLOOD LEVELS CAN BE MISLEADING

Proper electrolyte balance is essential to your life and well-being. Actually, it's so important that if the balance is significantly off, it can cause serious harm, or even death. People die every year from improper electrolyte concentration. Hyponatremia, which means low Sodium levels, and Hyperkalemia, which means high Potassium levels, individually or often in combination, are frequently seen in Emergency Room visits. You might imagine most of those patients are young athletes, sports players or hikers in hot weather, which absolutely can put you at risk for electrolyte imbalance, but in fact, many of these individuals tend to be older. As you age, your body becomes less able to naturally balance fluid and electrolytes. Because of their importance, you'd think monitoring Electrolytes in the CMP would be an essential health management strategy.

However, testing serum electrolyte levels is not actually a useful way to determine your true whole-body electrolyte status. While being "out of range" can indicate a serious issue, which is important to know and fix, being "in range" does not mean that your total body's stores of these minerals are adequate or optimal. So, why are serum electrolyte levels so misleading?

Your body tries to keep tight control of these minerals in your bloodstream because electrolytes are crucial for cell integrity, nerve signaling, and muscle function, which includes your heart and brain. So when the body senses blood electrolytes are low, it will steal minerals from other tissues to bring levels into a safe range. That means your blood levels might look fine, but your bones, organs, and muscles could be depleted of these minerals. This is why checking your blood electrolyte levels tells you very little about your nutritional status with regard to these minerals. By the time you see serum levels affected, your thinking, heart rate and muscle function can already be seriously impaired. So daily, common sense monitoring of symptoms and micronutrient nutrition/mineral intake are the best ways to evaluate your Electrolyte status. The common symptoms of electrolyte imbalances include: headaches, brain fog, irritability, dizziness, confusion, muscle cramps, poor sleep, and unexplained fatigue. At a mild to moderate level, these symptoms can be addressed through supplementation, but if you experience more severe symptoms seek medical attention.

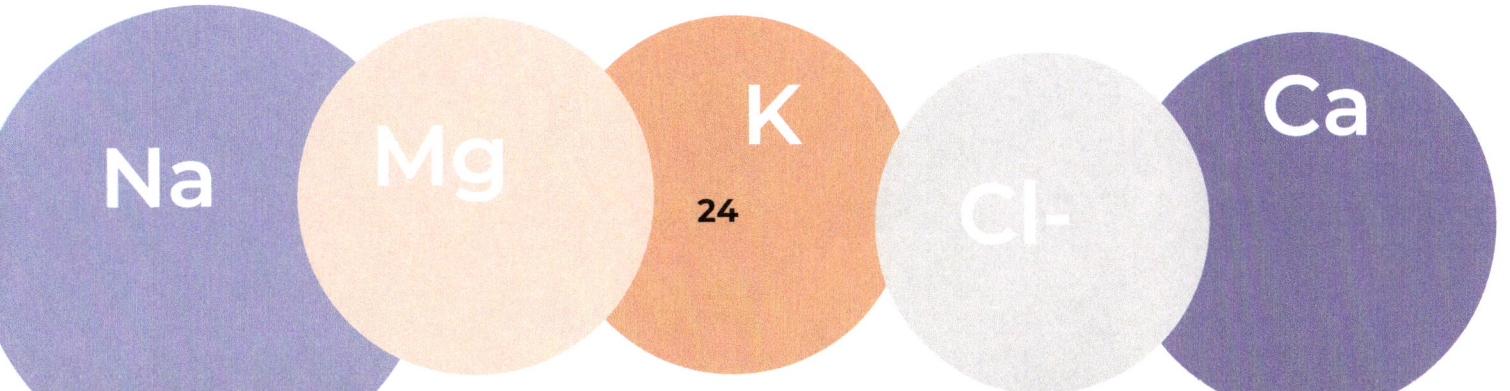

CBC w/ DIFF
(Complete Blood Count with Differential)

The CBC with Differential (sometimes listed as CBC w/Diff) looks at a detailed picture of the health of your Red and White Blood Cells (RBC and WBC) and Platelets. Compared to simply a CBC, a CBC w/Diff details the ratio each type of WBC, not just the total count. The term differential refers to differentiating the relative type of each WBC. By looking for abnormalities in different types of blood cells, your test results can alert you to possible infections, allergies, inflammation, or potentially even cancers. We can also get a peek at your hydration status, bone marrow health, and possible autoimmune issues.
.

When looking at a CBC w/Diff, your doctor is generally looking to see if anything is out of range. If any marker is out of range, your doctor will evaluate that in light of any known health conditions or medications that you may be taking.

For example, if your WBC count is slightly elevated, but you have a condition that leads to infection and inflammation, even something as small as an ingrown toenail, that would be a clear cause, and testing again once that issue is resolved would be beneficial. However, if there were no known or obvious causes, the out-of-range WBC count would require further investigation. Your doctor should suggest follow up tests to narrow down the source of the problem.

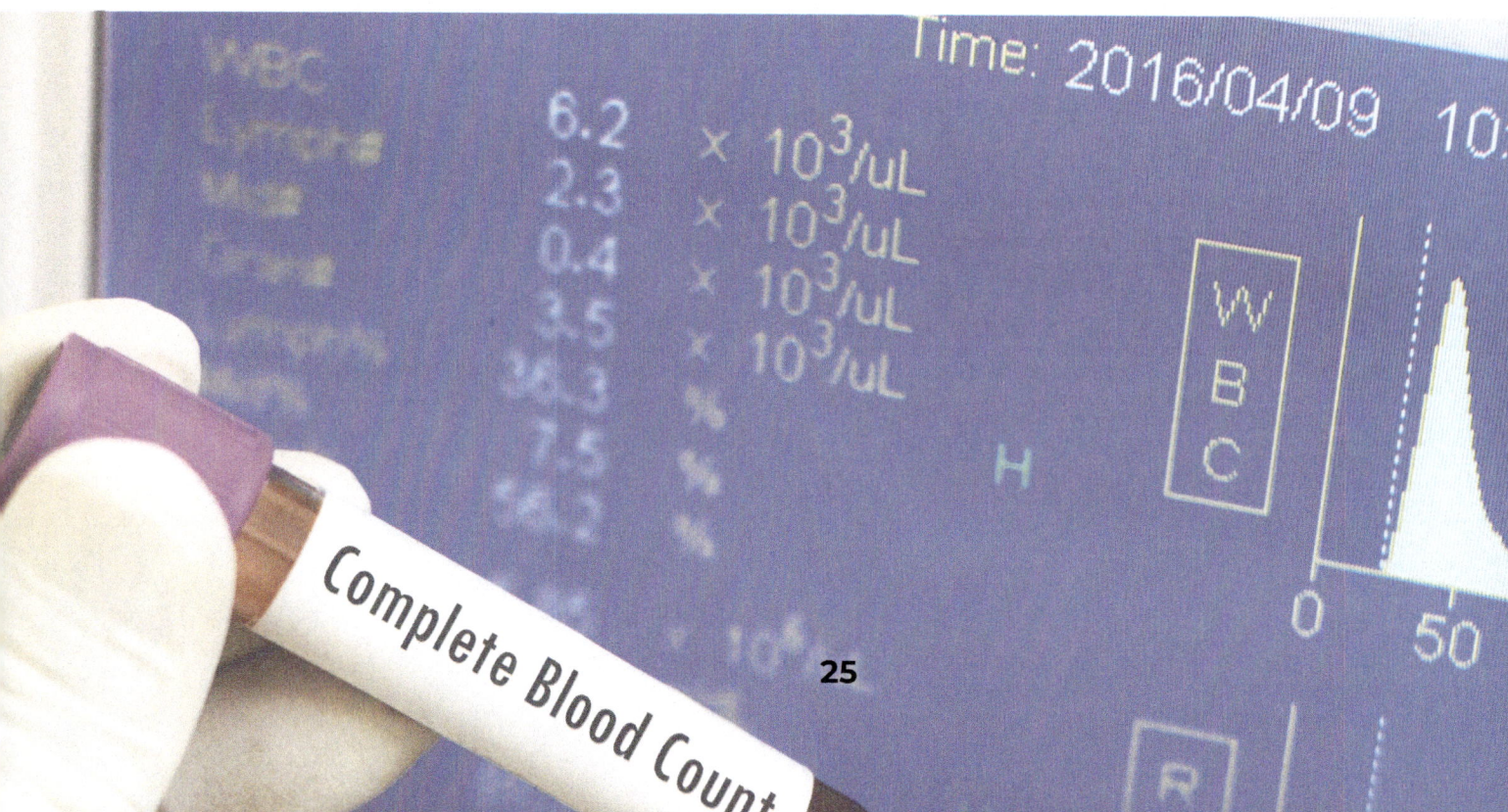

CBC with Diff
Here's What is Tested

Red Blood Cell Count is the measure of the RBC (red blood cells) density within a sample. The Hemoglobin in RBCs carries oxygen to tissues and organs. RBCs also help transport carbon dioxide out of the body. Low RBCs can suggest anemia or other problems. RBCs also interact with glucose, in a process called glycation – which is basically the process of glucose sticking to the Hemoglobin in RBCs. When glycation becomes excessive it impairs the function of the RBCs.

Hemoglobin is a protein molecule that is tasked with oxygen and carbon dioxide transport. Hemoglobin is what makes blood red. There can be variations in what is normal for each person based on gender, age, and fitness level.

Hematocrit is a measure of the volume percent of RBCs in the blood. While this percentage being off might indicate a health issue, it often points to an over or under-hydration issue as this affects the concentration of RBCs in blood volume.

Mean Corpuscular Volume (MCV) is a measure of the size of your RBCs. This can point to certain blood disorders or nutrient deficiencies, especially folic acid and vitamin B-12, and possibly iron.

Mean Corpuscular Hemoglobin (MCH) measures the amount of hemoglobin within a single Red Blood Cell. This most often points to anemia, or are looked at in conjunction with other tests to indicate wider health issues.

Mean Corpuscular Hemoglobin Concentration (MCHC) is similar to MCH but looks at the average concentration of hemoglobin. In addition to MCH, MCHC would also be looked at to evaluate anemia or other blood disorders.

Platelets are a necessary part of our blood as they are responsible for clotting as well as the transport of neurotransmitters and cytokines, cells that have an affect on the immune system. Small but mighty!

White Blood Cells (WBC) are a central part of the CBC w/Diff and there are a number of different types, which we'll explain in detail on the following page.

THE FIVE TYPES OF WHITE BLOOD CELLS

The 5 types of White Blood Cells (WBCs) each have a different role in a healthy body's immune system and in protecting against disease. When their numbers in your blood sample are higher than expected, this indicates your body is actively fighting something. Which type is elevated gives your doctor a clue into what that issue might be. Do not freak out if your WBCs are high in a test, it's a clue, not a confirmation of a serious problem. Stress or non-life threatening issues may be affecting numbers.

Neutrophils: These make up the majority of your WBCs, they are first on the scene to confront infection. Neutrophils target bacteria and fungi. They are highly mobile and move freely through the body.

Lymphocytes: There are three types of Lymphocytes - B cells, T cells, and NK cells. These are made from stem cells in the bone marrow. B cells make antibodies to target antigens, which are foreign substances which triggers the immune system. T and NK cells attack virus-infected and cancer cells.

Basophils: These cells predominantly fight parasitic infection, limit blood clotting and release histamine in response to allergic reactions.

Eosinophils: This component of our immune system fights off infections and pathogens. As part of the allergy reaction cycle, too high a level of eosinophils might be indicative of an over-reactive immune system.

Monocytes: As the largest type of WBC, they are capable of attacking foreign cells as well as infected host cells.

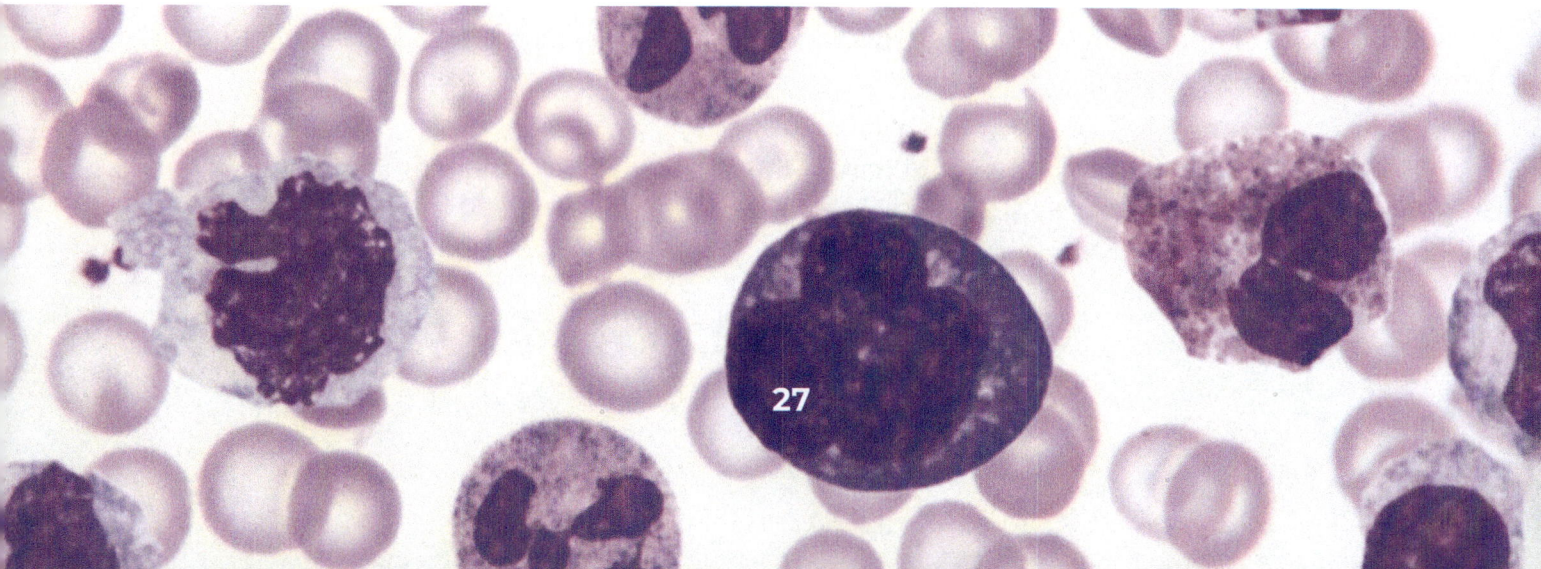

WHAT'S IN A BASIC LIPID PANEL?

Once upon a time doctors erroneously based everything about heart health on your LDL being in or out of range. Oh wait, that's still happening now. As medical research advances, it takes quite a while for doctors to catch wind of the changes. One of those changes is our understanding of how lipids affect our heart disease risk.

A Lipid panel, in simple terms, looks at fats within the body, there are a variety of these, most notably cholesterol and triglycerides. Lipids are complex, but confusingly, we are led to believe that they are simple. Because of the true complexity, we want to give you a brief overview, but with the common sense understanding that this book will only touch the surface of these compounds.

Cholesterol is a type of lipid called a sterol that actually has a number of functions. Around 75% of the cholesterol in your body is produced by the liver, the rest comes from food. Cholesterol is essential to life; it's required for sex hormone production, cell membrane integrity, and bile production. What is often referred to in the lipid panel as cholesterol is not solely cholesterol, it is a "package" of a lipid plus a protein, called a Lipoprotein.

In a basic Lipid Panel, you'll most often see LDL, HDL, Triglycerides, and sometimes VLDL.

LDL: Low-Density Lipoprotein. These have a larger proportion of cholesterol to protein, making them less dense. LDL is the package that carries cholesterol (and many other useful things) to the cells for use. You will sometimes hear this erroneously called "Bad" Cholesterol.

HDL: High-Density Lipoprotein. These have a larger proportion of protein to cholesterol, making them denser. HDL is the package that returns cholesterol to the liver for recycling.
You will sometimes hear this referred to as "Good" Cholesterol.

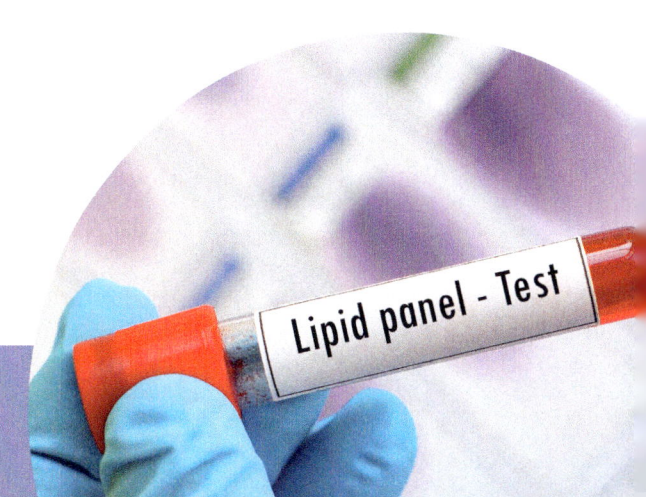

WHAT ELSE IS IN A BASIC LIPID PANEL?

Total Cholesterol: This is a calculation of your HDL, LDL, and VLDL (Very Low-Density Lipoproteins). Because of its non-specific nature, it's not extremely useful. While this calculation can be of interest as data on a population level, a good doctor won't base their diagnosis or plan health decisions solely on total cholesterol.

Triglycerides: also known as "Trigs" are named for their structure, three fatty acids with a glycerol backbone. Triglycerides are the main lipid in the blood, and if they are at exceedingly high levels in a sample, they can give it surprisingly cloudy or milky appearance. This is not a scenario you want!

The primary driver of chronic high triglycerides is consumption of too much energy, especially in the form of carbohydrates/sugars. High triglycerides are correlated to one of the biggest threats to your good health, Metabolic Syndrome.

As we will discuss in a bit, to get a good picture of metabolic health you'll want to know your Trigs and HDL. Surprisingly, not important in the picture of Metabolic Health markers is LDL. If you want to truly understand LDL and its relationship to cardiovascular health, that's a course in and of itself. A basic Lipid Panel in isolation is insufficient to seriously evaluate cardiovascular risk.

Truly understanding the relationship of LDL to heart disease is beyond an introductory topic. If this is an area of real concern for you, you'll want to consider a deeper inquiry by learning about things like particle patterns, ApoB, and risk scores rather than making decisions on incomplete information like LDL alone.

If you are someone with specific coronary concerns and want to dive further into a few resources:
Some of our favorite voices on Cholesterol are Dave Feldman and Siobhan Huggins at CholesterolCode.com, Bret Scher, MD at lowcarbcardiologist.com (these two are especially useful if on a low-carb eating approach), and for a perspective on lipids that, while we aren't always in agreement with, we always feel enriched by the discussion at: PeterAttiaMD.com

INDIVIDUAL TESTS: TESTING A LA CARTE

So far we've detailed the Lab Panels in the Annual Labs list. On the following pages, we will cover the individual tests Dr. Berry recommends. Adding these individual tests rounds out the basic annual checkup for that hypothetical average patient who is symptom-free, and wants a baseline health check.

Occasionally some folks say they are shocked that this list isn't much longer. There are sometimes great reasons to run more tests... when they are conditionally appropriate. But throwing dozen of tests at the patient, that are unnecessary for most of you, would be a disservice. Too often we see practitioners who order many obscure and unnecessary tests, and are really just looking for ways to sell supplement packages.

Your doctor may suggest a few additional labs for you that we don't list here. That's awesome! Within the general population, there will always be some variation. This is the list Dr. Berry starts with for everyone coming into the clinic in apparent good health.

THE INDIVIDUAL TESTS: EXPLAINED

B-12	Also known as cobalamin, it is a vitamin essential to Red Blood Cell formation, nerve function, and cell metabolism. Deficiency can lead to anemia, exhaustion, muscle weakness, and nerve dysfunction.
C-Peptide	A proxy measure that indicates average insulin levels. Insulin is produced connected to a C-peptide molecule, hence C for connected. in response to carbohydrate intake. This test is important because tracking C-Peptide can prevent future diabetes.
Copper	An essential mineral that plays a role in the regulation of iron metabolism, nervous system function, connective tissue creation, energy production, and melanin.
DHEA-S	(Dehydroepiandrosterone Sulfate) A hormone present in both sexes, in varying amounts. This test evaluates adrenal function and hormonal balance.
ESR	Also known as SED Rate, this is a test of inflammation. This test looks at the rate of sedimentation from RBCs in a sample. A high rate can indicate an issue with inflammation in the body.
Ferritin	A blood protein related to Iron levels. Specifically, it looks at Iron storage in the blood, compared to baseline levels of Iron. High Ferritin levels tend to be seen in inflammatory reactions. Low Ferritin can mean your body's ability to access Iron is impaired.

THE INDIVIDUAL TESTS: EXPLAINED

GGT	(Gamma-Glutamyl Transferase) An enzyme found throughout the body, but mostly in the liver. An out-of-range number indicates liver or bile duct damage. Taken in context with the other liver tests, a clinician can incorporate this reading when assessing overall liver health.

hbA1c

(Hemoglobin A1c) Measures glycation of the red blood cells (RBCs), glycation refers to glucose molecules attached to the hemoglobin, which is a protein in red blood cells. A small amount of glycation is normal and expected, but too much generally indicates problems with your blood sugar concentration. hbA1c is often shortened to just A1C.

Current medical guidelines have A1C as the diagnostic tool to confirm diabetes, as it generally gives us the average blood glucose, and in fact is often referred to as eAG - estimated average glucose. The A1C is useful as rather than simply showing a snapshot in time, such as with a fasting glucose number, it calculates this estimated average glucose over a longer span of 3 months. We agree folks should be monitoring A1C, but there are a few caveats to be aware of:

Because the calculation on A1C depends on the average lifespan and size of an RBC, if an individual has shorter or longer living RBCs, which might happen on low carb or carnivore diets, or larger or smaller RBCs, as with genetic conditions like beta-thalassemia, this can skew the results. Anemia is another condition that can affect A1C. In a recent study, about 33% of the participants had RBC lifespans that fell outside the standardized lifespan range. If your A1C is unexpectedly out of range, you may be part of that 33%. and there are a few tests such as Fructosamine and/or Glycated Albumin (GA) that can deliver better estimates on average blood glucose.

Homocysteine	An amino acid that serves as a precursor molecule for a number of other compounds in the body. High levels can cause blood clots and cardiovascular damage and can be an indication of a Vitamin B deficiency.

THE INDIVIDUAL TESTS: EXPLAINED

hs-CRP	(high sensitivity C Reactive Protein, where C stands for Carbohydrate antigen) While often misunderstood as being specifically related to only cardiac issues, this test is actually a non-specified marker of inflammation. Though it can be cardiac related, it is often high high due to other inflammation sources such as autoimmune issues, injury, or illness. Because of its non-specific nature, follow-up on high readings is always indicated. Make sure you are testing hs-CRP, not simple CRP as that test is not sensitive enough to deliver useful information.
Insulin, Fasting	One of the central tests for diagnosing hyperinsulinemia, which strongly suggests metabolic syndrome. Our bodies need a base amount of insulin to function properly, however, that level is a relatively low number. When fasting insulin levels are high it indicates that the body is overproducing insulin, which can be very damaging on a long-term basis.
Iron	A crucial mineral that serves several functions. Iron is part of hemoglobin, keeping our blood and muscles oxygenated. Iron is also part of many other proteins and enzymes, and levels are kept tightly controlled. Too little risks anemia, which impairs the RBCs ability to carry enough oxygen, but too much can be toxic.
Magnesium	An electrolyte crucial for muscle function and proper sleep. Most of us are likely to be Magnesium deficient. Low levels can cause anxiety, insomnia, muscle cramps, constipation, poor glucose regulation and sometimes cardiac arrythmia.
Phosphorus	A electrolyte/mineral that is vital in nerve function as well as bone health. Low levels are caused by nutritional deficiencies and can result in muscle weakness and poor bone strength, which can cause fractures, while high levels might be caused by liver or kidney filtration/excretion problems.

THE INDIVIDUAL TESTS: EXPLAINED

TSH — (Thyroid Stimulating Hormone) A hormone produced in the pituitary in response to the body's supply of thyroid hormone. A TSH can be used to check if your body seems to be producing enough thyroid hormones. This test is sufficient if you are non-symptomatic, however if you have symptoms you'd want to be sure to check additional thyroid markers (see page 44) and not rely solely on a TSH for diagnosis.

Uric Acid — Uric acid is a waste product of purine breakdown, spurred by the overconsumption of fructose and alcohol. Though purines are also found in organ meat and shellfish we do not believe those are a direct cause of high Uric acid in healthy individuals. Even in the absence of overconsumption of these, those with Metabolic Syndrome will generally have high Uric Acid levels.

We find that as people become more Metabolically healthy, Uric Acid levels reduce naturally. Additionally, poor thyroid function can impair Uric Acid excretion, and certain vitamin deficiencies, especially Vitamin C, can also cause high Uric Acid.

Urinalysis — A simple check-in to confirm that urine does not contain things it should not. Urine should be light yellow (barring any vitamin ingestion that affects color), with a clear, not cloudy appearance, and there should not be traces of protein or blood. Ketones are also measured, and while the testing parameters suggests you want to be negative for ketones, when someone is on a low carbohydrate diet, the presence of ketones is normal.

Vitamin C — Also known as ascorbic acid, required to form blood vessels, cartilage, muscle, and collagen. Vital to heal wounds properly, as well as avoid deficiency-related diseases such as scurvy. Low Vitamin C can also cause elevated Uric Acid levels.

THE INDIVIDUAL TESTS: EXPLAINED

Vitamin D (25)	Vitamin D levels are essential to immune function, as well as cell and bone health, mood, wound healing and kidney function. There are several tests, make sure to get the D 25 test, as other tests can be inaccurate. This specific test measures Vitamin D in your blood once it's been converted to the usable form.
Zinc	A trace mineral that is required for enzyme function. Plays a role in the creation of DNA, growth of cells, building proteins, healing damaged tissue, and supporting a healthy immune system.

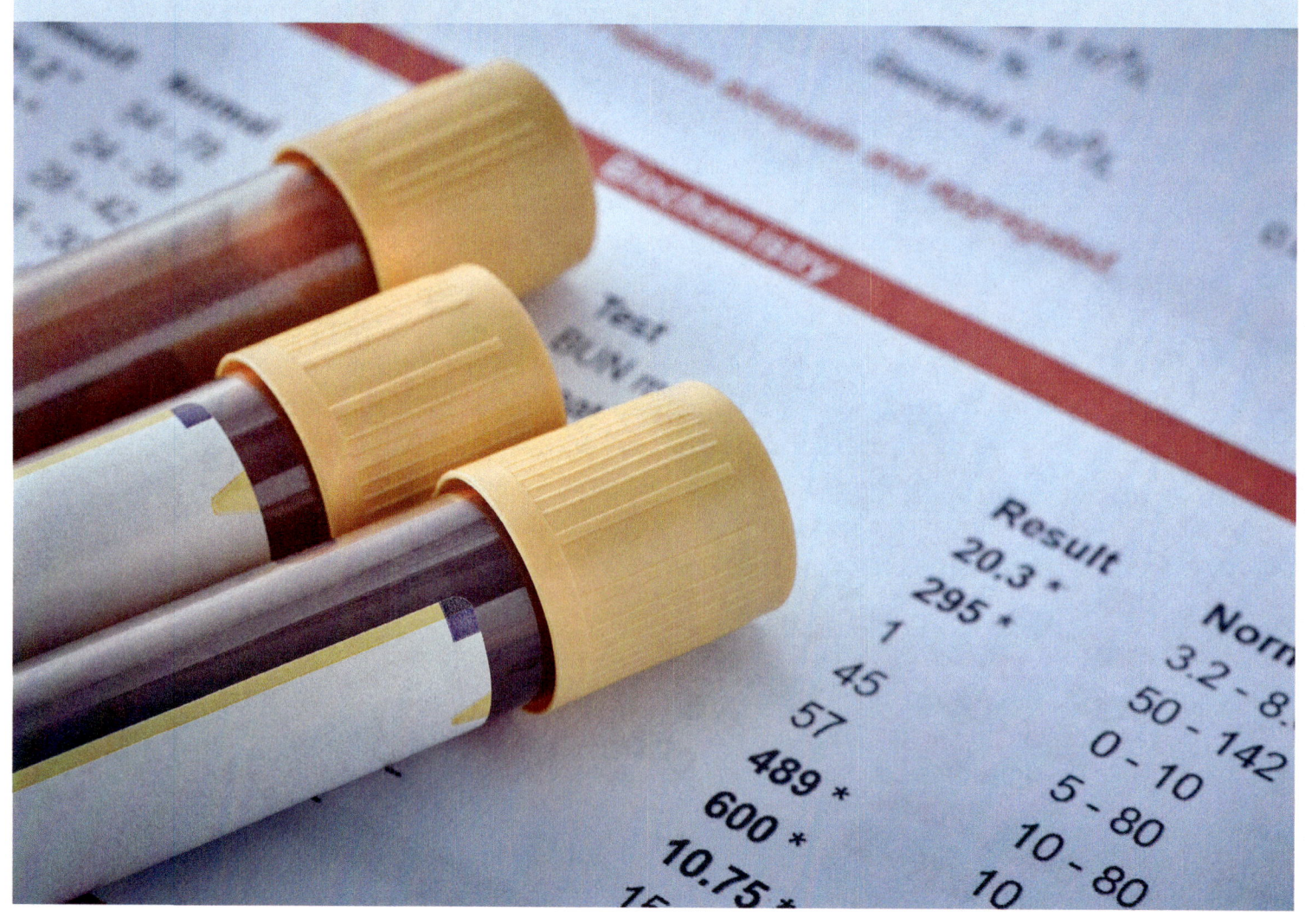

SUSIE'S BLOOD SUGAR

For the past five years, when Susie went for her annual physical, they always ran a CBC. As her glucose was always between 95 and 99 mg/dL on that panel, every year her doctor told her everything looked great and he'd see her next year.

At this year's physical, she joked that it was time for new glasses as her vision was getting worse. When they ran the blood work this time, they found that her fasting glucose was over 100 mg/dL and the doctor decided to do a follow-up lab - the A1c.

They were shocked when it came back to 11%! Susie's blood sugar was not just a little high - she was deeply diabetic! And that blurry vision wasn't from aging - it was damage to the blood vessels in her eyes from chronic high blood sugar.

Turns out, that even though Susie's glucose reading skirted under the problem line, she'd been first pre-diabetic, then advanced to full-blown diabetic without anyone picking it up. That is because no one ran additional tests to check her blood sugar or insulin levels beyond that one daily snapshot of her fasting glucose.

Glucose levels change minute by minute. It's entirely possible for someone's glucose problems to be disguised because it just so happened that one day was a good one in terms of glucose control. But 99% of the rest of the time, the number might not have been so rosy. (The reverse is also possible, a night of bad sleep can make you look diabetic the next day, but it's not a persistent issue.)

Because Susie's condition was allowed to progress unchecked for so long, her vision is now permanently damaged. The eye is filled with tiny blood vessels that will never recover from those highs she was experiencing.

If her doctor had been running A1c's all those years, which show an average of your glucose, not just a snapshot, this would have been caught. And Susie could still drive at night.

Unfortunately, this story is all too common. There were several signs such as rising C-peptide, Insulin, and A1c. Any of those blood tests would have raised a red flag in time to save her from the lifetime of dealing with the damage caused.

For some, that damage might be to their eyes, others - the kidneys, and still others - the heart. Chronic high blood sugar is a killer, and you don't want to rely on the hope that you'll be a lucky one who doesn't have long-term consequences.

COMMON SENSE METABOLIC MATTERS

A central focus of our recommendations (Kim as a Coach and Ken as a Doctor) revolve around improving metabolic health. Within the Annual Labs list, we've shared several markers that will help you monitor where you stand with some metabolic markers.

Getting and staying metabolically healthy is the best investment a person can make to improve their long-term health. But as we mentioned earlier, 88% of Americans fall short of meeting all the criteria of being metabolically healthy. (Arujo, et al., 2019)

In the analysis that determined this shockingly low rate of metabolic health, they defined the parameters of metabolic health as:

BLOOD PRESSURE	FASTING BLOOD GLUCOSE / A1C	TRIGS	HDL	WAIST MEASURE*
120/80 mm/Hg or lower	<100 mg/dL / 5.7%	<150 mg/dL	>50 mg/dL (Women) >40 mg/dL (Men)	<34.6" (WOMEN) <40" (MEN)

We actually think some of these markers are a bit too generous. We'd prefer to see Trigs <100 mg/dL and A1c under 5.4%.

Plus, we'd add some additional markers to that:

C-Peptide: Very Good: between 0.5 to 1.99 ng/dL / Optimal: 0.5 to 1.7 ng/dL
Fasting Insulin: Very Good: 2 to 8 IU/mL / Optimal: 5 IU/mL or under

We've added these tests as they sum up a lot of metabolic activity, and dysregulation can show up earlier in these markers before you see the effects appear in blood sugar or blood pressure measurements. We firmly believe that the sooner the intervention, the easier it will be to fix, and the less long-term damage will be done.

WAIST WHERE?

We recommend defining the waist as the midpoint between your ribs and the top of your hipbone, so to find this, feel for the soft gap on your side between your ribs and hips and find the middle point (on many this is their narrowest abdominal measure). We also think using a hard number for waist cut-offs regardless of height, as they did in the analysis, has issues, and suggest instead evaluating your waist-to-height ratio instead.
That waist-to-height ratio should be .5 or lower. So if you are 60" tall, you want your waist to be no larger than 30"

You'll often hear the advice to measure the waist at the belly button, but if your abdomen has ever been stretched (pregnancy, extreme weight gain, etc) Your belly button may have drifted several inches lower and will no longer be an accurate guide. This is why we recommend skeletal guideposts instead.

C-PEPTIDE & FASTING INSULIN

C-peptide is a proxy measurement of how much insulin your body is producing.

Your body produces a molecule of C-peptide for every molecule of Insulin, therefore you can track C-peptide and it will give you an approximation of your average insulin production.

Proxy Measurement: Something that can be measured directly as an indirect measure of another marker.

Fasting Insulin is simply testing the amount of insulin in your body in the fasted state. The assumption is that after an overnight fast, your insulin has now fallen to its basal, or low base level.

Therefore, when we look at both, we should have a view of your basal (baseline) level of insulin and how much it fluctuates over the day.

HOW IMPORTANT IS METABOLIC HEALTH?

Since you are reading this book, hopefully, you know the answer to this: VERY!

We also want to emphasize that change takes time. If your numbers aren't yet optimal, just seek improvement over time! Target ranges are a goal you can aim towards, but should never be something you beat yourself up about not achieving yet.

In terms of metabolic health, even a 10% improvement in body composition can yield huge health benefits. That might be a tiny fraction of your overall goals, but the body loves improvements and will reward you with significant disease risk reduction. Just get started and keep going!

The goal is Progress, not Perfection.

So many of our patients and clients look at metrics like these markers and throw their hands up because they feel so far from them. We are here to tell you, that's dumb.
Human and understandable, but dumb.

We get it. We can be dumb too.
But good friends are the ones who tell you when you need to snap out of it! Don't let your expectations get in the way of improvement!

Section 3:
Labs to Check When You Have Symptoms

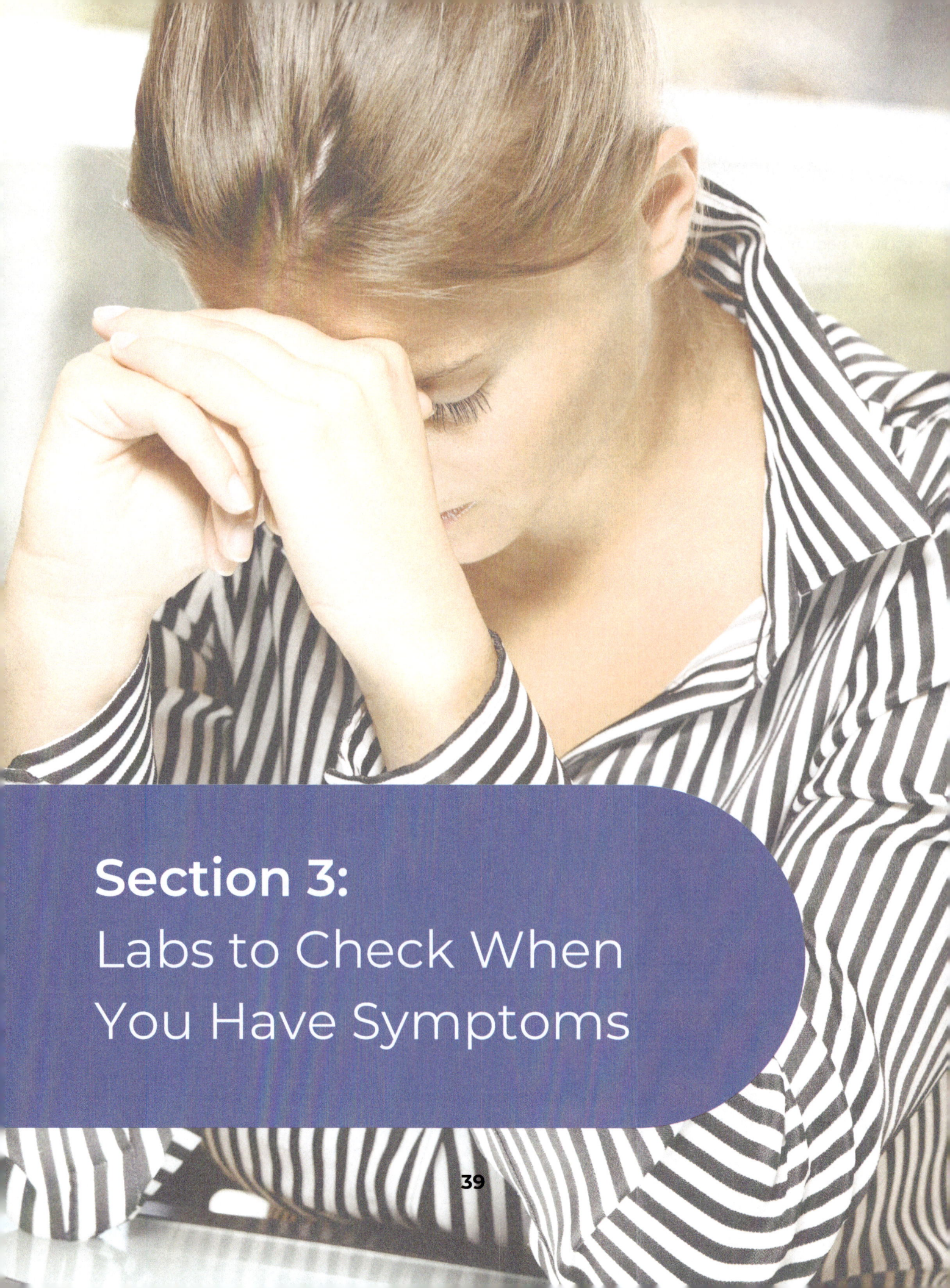

Now you know which tests should be run annually for a person who is in reasonably good health and living a fairly complaint-free life. Well, in terms of health and symptoms that is!

But what if you are not symptom-free? What if you suffer from some common issues that folks write off as "just getting old" or some other such nonsense?
What should you do then?

Level 2:
BUT WHAT IF I AM NOT SYMPTOM-FREE?

In the scope of this book, it is impossible for us to describe **ALL** possible symptoms and/or illnesses. If we went into all that detail this book would be 50,000 pages long and come with a medical degree. It would be improper, and frankly, irresponsible to suggest that this little book can approach being a comprehensive medical tool.

However, we felt it was important to discuss some incredibly common (and fairly straightforward) conditions/issues that are not thoroughly investigated by the average doctor and some common diagnoses that are used as a catch-all when a doctor is too time-starved (or too lazy) to look into, though they should.
If you don't find your symptom/situation listed here, it doesn't mean it shouldn't be investigated. You will simply need a custom, in-person approach.

The reality is, most folks seeking out medical advice are not in super great health and symptom-free. It's human nature not to want to address problems preemptively. So, if you are one of the many folks who are saying, "But I DO have symptoms," or "I just don't feel normal," read on. Let's start with a definition.

We throw that word around all the time – Symptom. What does that even mean?

A symptom is any physical/mental manifestation of not-quite-rightness that can be indicative of disease.

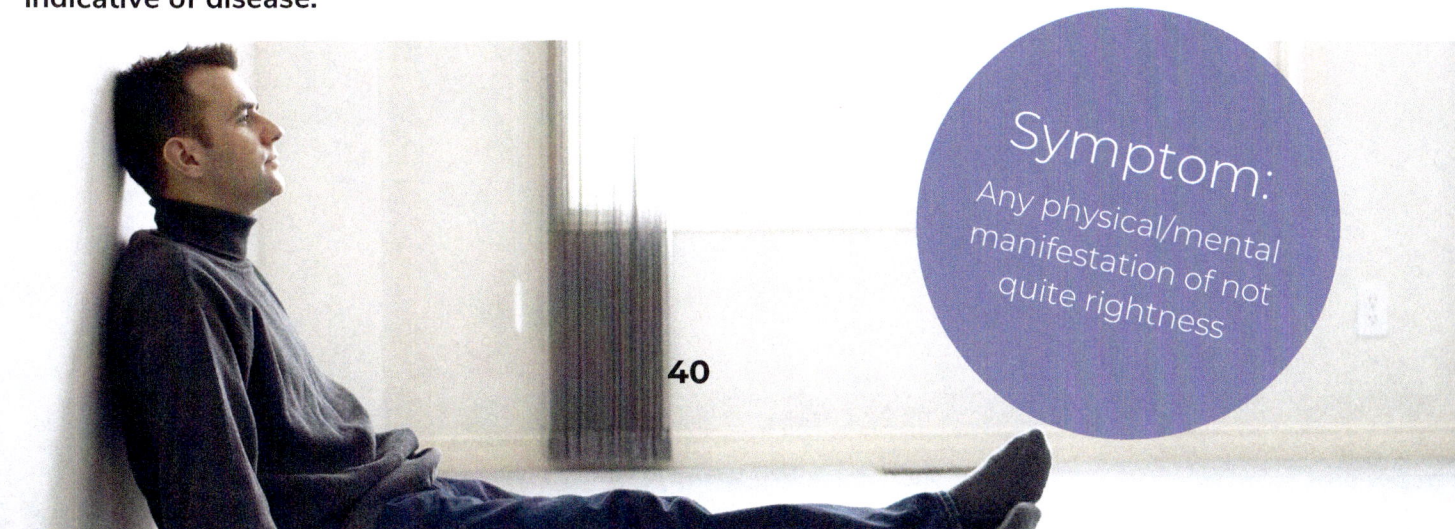

Symptom: Any physical/mental manifestation of not quite rightness

COMMONLY REPORTED SYMPTOMS:

- Tired/Fatigue/Weakness: This includes feeling exhausted, a general malaise, can't quite wake up, constantly wanting a nap, feeling overwhelmed, feeling under-fueled

- Anxiety/Unexplained Emotional Fluctuations/Sadness

- Can't Lose Weight/Unexplained Weight Gain or Loss

- General or specific Gastric Distress including Abdominal Pain

- Brain Fog/Forgetfulness

- Low Libido/Sex Drive

- Headaches/Chronic Migraines

- Hair Loss

- Bodily Aches and Pains

- Lack of Motivation/Low Energy

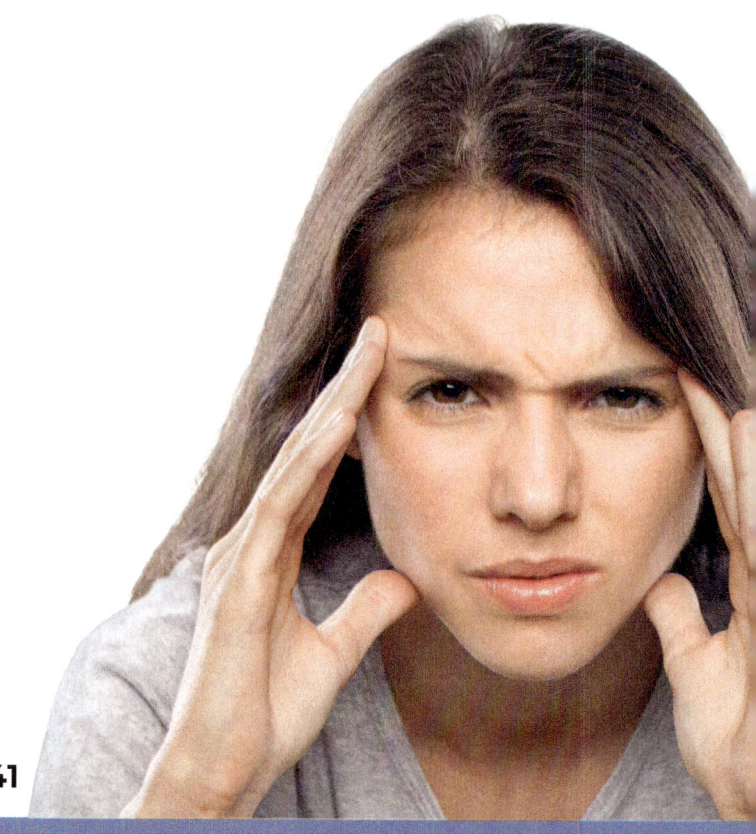

MASTER HORMONES & SYSTEMS

In terms of health, there are a few body systems that tend to be implicated in a majority of health issues. Hormonal systems (especially the thyroid), chronic inflammatory processes, and nutrient deficiencies are almost always the first things to look at when symptoms arise.

Now, don't get us wrong - these are not always simple things to fix (though some are!), but there are simple blood tests to run that can give incredible insight into what might be going wrong. While these certainly aren't always the culprit, they are good to rule out before proceeding to more complex possibilities.

When Patients present with symptoms, these are the areas that almost always warrant consideration and thorough investigation.

The first two were investigated in labs within the Annual Labs in section 1:

- **Specific Nutrient Deficiencies**
- **Immunological Markers/Acute Phase Reactants**

Beyond that, the most comon areas that need investigating are usually:

- **Thyroid**
- **Sex Hormones**

Plus we add one more test, not because it is most common, but because it is so often overlooked:

- **Parathyroid**

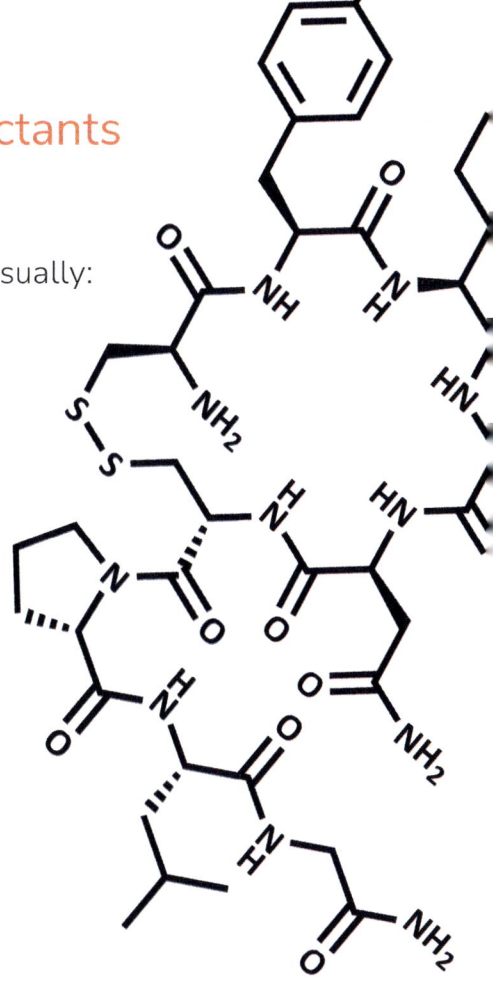

SYMPTOMS & TESTING REFERENCE SHEET

Use this chart to identify common lab tests to investigate as a starting place when evaluating possible causes depending on your specific symptoms.

INVESTIGATE	SYMPTOMS
Full Thyroid Panel	Fatigue, Foggy Headed, Unexplained Weight Gain or Loss, Disturbed Sleep, Libido Issues, Hair Loss, Headaches, Abdominal Pain, Mood Changes, Body Aches & Pain
CMP	Fatigue, Unexplained Weight Gain or Loss
Sex Hormone Panel	Fatigue, Unexplained Weight Gain or Loss, Disturbed Sleep, Libido Issues, Hair Loss, Headaches, Mood Changes, Body Aches and Pains
Complete Blood Count (CBC)	Fatigue, Unexplained Weight Gain or Loss, Disturbed Sleep, Libido Issues, Hair Loss, Headaches, Abdominal Pain, Mood Changes, Body Aches & Pain
Insulin, Serum & C-peptide	Fatigue, Unexplained Weight Gain or Loss, Libido, Hair Loss, Mood Changes, Body Aches & Pain
Calcium	Abdominal Pain, Mood Changes, Body Aches & Pain, Kidney Stones
Homocysteine	Body Aches, Pain, Inflammation. Overweight
Ferritin	Body Aches, Pain, Foggy Headed, Fatigue, Inflammation. Overweight
hs-CRP	Body Aches, Pain, Inflammation. Overweight
ESR (sed rate)	Body Aches, Pain, Inflammation. Overweight
Iron, Serum	Body Aches, Pain Foggy Headed, Fatigue
hbA1c	Body Aches, Pain, Weight Issues, Repeated Infections
Amylase & Lipase	Unexplained Abdominal Pain
Magnesium	Fatigue, Unexplained Weight Gain or Loss, Body Aches & Pain
Zinc	Fatigue, Unexplained Weight Gain or Loss, Body Aches & Pain, Repeated Infections
Vitamin D 25	Fatigue, Unexplained Weight Gain or Loss, Body Aches & Pain, Repeated Infections

ALL ABOUT THE THYROID

The thyroid is a butterfly-shaped gland at the base of the throat. We've seen an epidemic of thyroid problems in recent years. While the majority of cases of thyroid problems seem to occur in women, they also occur in men. Most doctors will only test one specific number - TSH or Thyroid Stimulating Hormone, and if that's in range it's pronounced that the patient's thyroid is "fine." However, the reality is TSH is a test that misses the majority of problems. Some doctors will also test T4, which also falls far short of testing needs.

Thyroid issues tend to fall into either Hypo or Hyper type of defect. Hypothyroid indicates lower than required thyroid function. Hyperthyroidism indicates an overactive thyroid. Both are of significant concern, though hypothyroidism is far more common than hyperthyroidism. In general, hypothyroidism causes a significantly slowed metabolism, while hyperthyroidism causes a significantly increased rate and eventually leads to the breakdown of the thyroid, which then can result in hypothyroidism.

To get a better understanding of what needs to be tested, let's look at the specific markers of thyroid function to get a better understanding of why we need to be more comprehensive in our investigation.

The list of tests one should run for a full thyroid panel is:

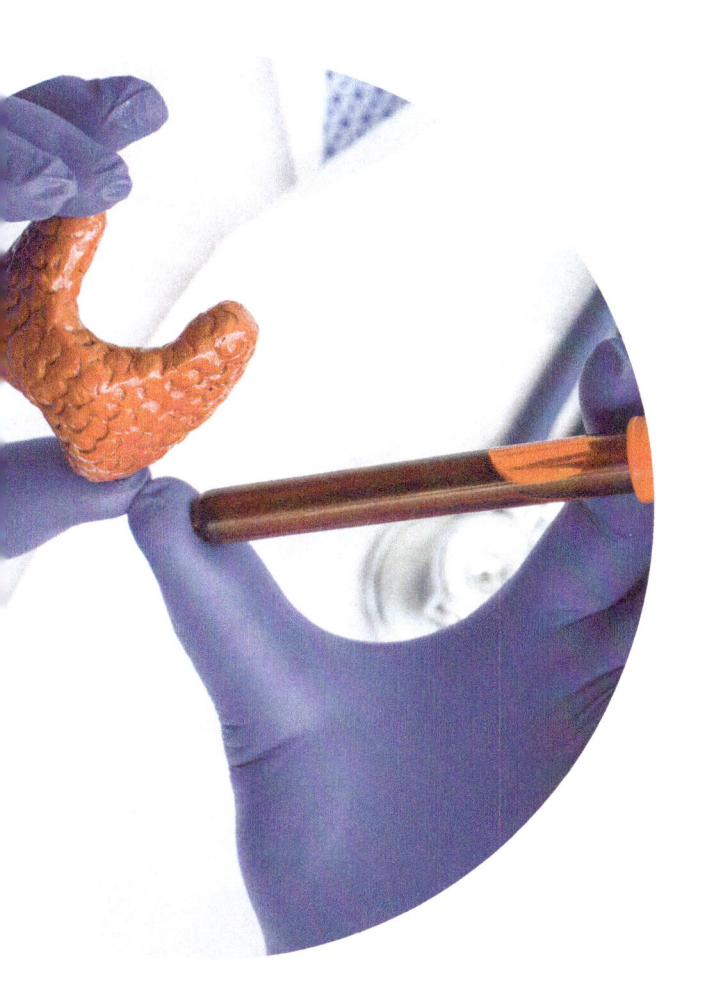

THE TESTS

- **TSH (Thyroid Stimulating Hormone)**
- **T4, free (Thyroxine)**
- **T3, Free (Triiodothyronine)**
- **T3 Reverse**
- **Thyroid Peroxidase Antibodies**
- **Thyroglobulin Antibodies**

AN OVERVIEW OF THE THYROID

Before we go further, let's get an overview of the Thyroid microcosm to understand how all these elements interact. T4 (thyroxine) is the primary thyroid hormone produced by the thyroid gland. It has 4 atoms of iodine, hence T4.

Inside our brain, there's a gland called the pituitary, inside of which we produce a hormone called TSH – thyroid-stimulating hormone. As our body seeks to maintain proper balance, there's an ongoing conversation between TSH, T3 and T4. More TSH is secreted if the body senses T3 and T4 is low, and less is secreted if they seems high. People can easily get confused by TSH because high TSH means low Thyroid function and vice versa, which seems counter-intuitive. But that is because TSH is a stimulating hormone - so a high TSH means your body is signaling for increased release.

Thyroid hormones are found in the body in both bound and unbound forms as they bind to carrier proteins for transport; the bound form is unavailable for use, as it's bound to a protein.

Due to other hormone fluctuations, these carrier proteins can vary in concentration, making the unbound form a better gauge in general, when testing available thyroid levels.

Total T4 reflects the total amount of T4, both bound and unbound.
Free T4 is just the amount of T4 that is not bound to carrier proteins, and therefore it is free in the bloodstream and available for use.
T4 is a mostly inactive hormone – meaning it must be converted to the active form – T3 (which it does by giving up one iodine atom) for it to be used by the body.

T3 is also found in both bound and unbound forms.

THYROXINE is the primary thyroid hormone produced by the body. It has 4 atoms

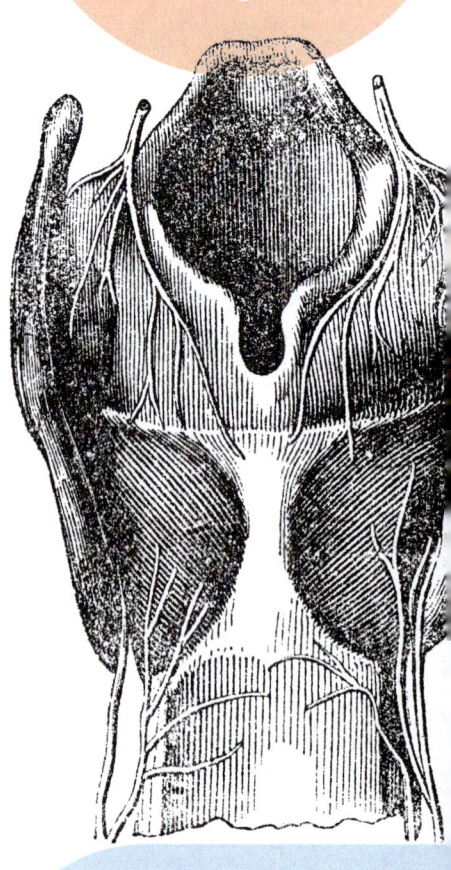

T4 is an inactive hormone

As T4 is converted to T3 through the removal of an outer iodine atom, reverse T3 can be created when that iodine atom ends up in the wrong location.

Reverse T3 (RT3) is a biologically inactive metabolite. Reverse T3 can be high due to many issues – both short-term illnesses, long-term conditions, poor nutrition/nutrient deficiencies/chronic under-eating as well as diseases and/or medicines. In the absence of these issues, it can simply be seen as an indicator of poor T4 to T3 conversion.

Some doctors will order actually order free T4 and T3, but still totally miss Reverse T3. Reverse T3 is a detail that is imperative, as it is the best way to see a very common problem - when there is poor T4 to T3 conversion. This problem is especially common in cases of metabolic issues.

One can have good TSH and good T4 numbers, but high RT3 - it's sort of like your packages got delivered, so Amazon says your order is complete but they delivered them to the empty house next door. It's delivered, but you can't access it or use it.

Lastly on our list of tests are two tests to evaluate Thyroid Antibodies – Thyroid Peroxidase (TPO) and Thyroglobulin Antibodies (TGaB). These antibodies are produced when the body mistakenly targets the thyroid hormones as invaders and mounts an immune response to the thyroid.

The presence of these antibodies indicates that some degree of the auto-immune condition, Hashimoto's Thyroiditis, is present and acting in a hostile manner towards the thyroid gland.
If positive for Hashimoto's thyroiditis (often called just Hashimoto's or Hashi's for short) the goal is to get and keep the antibody count as low as possible, as continued high antibodies indicate the immune system is still attacking the gland. Some are able to keep those levels vary low to undetectable, and some consider this being "in remission"in terms of this autoimmune condition.

A note on testing - some women find their thyroid levels fluctuate through their menstrual cycle due to changes in sex hormones. At mid-cycle, TSH may be elevated. Keep this in mind when comparing labs done at different times in your cycle. Additionally, TSH can vary depending on time of day or in response to heavy exercise prior to testing due to TSH's energy-sensing role.

WHY IS PROPER THYROID FUNCTION SO IMPORTANT?

Many of us only think of the thyroid as important to metabolism - aka energy utilization. But thyroid function is involved in so many body processes- it is essential to life. You literally can't survive without thyroid hormones. If your thyroid is removed or damaged, you must supplement. Proper thyroid hormones help us regulate body temperature, mood, blood pressure, immune function, brain and mood health, metabolic issues, growth of skin, hair, bone, muscle, and more.

Notably, glucose uptake into brain and muscle tissue are aided by healthy thyroid function as well as bone mineral density. These functions are essential to healthy aging and maintaining good blood sugar management.

What are the causes of thyroid problems? There can absolutely be some nutrient deficiencies or reactivity that, if fixed, may reverse the thyroid malfunction. As mentioned previously, most cases of hypothyroidism seem to be caused by Hashimoto's. Other autoimmune issues may also be implicated in causes, as well as an overall issue with metabolic health.

For others with thyroid issues, they remain idiopathic - that is - we are unclear on the cause. Even if never reversed, with proper supplementation, these folks can live very healthy lives.

Now that we have a picture of how the main thyroid hormones interact, we can see some of the places the process breaks down. You might make plenty of T4, but it is remaining in the bound form, and is not being freed up to freeform, so not enough is available to convert to T3 in proper amounts. But if you'd only tested total T4, you'd have missed that. Or you might be making lots of T3, but too much of it is going to reverse T3, and not available for metabolic needs.

You can see how easily thyroid problems can become a terrible state of "water water everywhere, but not a drop to drink."

THYROID NOTES
Thyroid Supplementation

While we won't go deeply into medications and supplements here in this book, we do feel moved to point out a few things.

The most commonly prescribed thyroid medication is Synthroid. As its name would indicate, it's synthetic T4. Fake T4 and JUST T4. And as we discussed above, a very common issue is impaired T4 to T3 conversion. For many folks, using T4-only supplementation is like pouring a cup of water into the ocean.

We really suggest everyone look into using natural desiccated thyroid (NDT) supplementation - which is a measured dose of animal thyroid hormone, which automatically contains T3 and T4, so if your issue is one of conversion, you'll gain a benefit from taking the supplement including the already converted form. Countless patients experience incredible benefits by switching to this form.
However, it's important to track your symptoms and how you feel and function in response to medication. While some forms work for most folks, we do see individual differences and it pays off to work with your doctor to tinker with both dosage and possibly the maker of the meds until you feel optimized. There are some folks who need a more custom blend of T4 and T3 rather than the standard ratio available in NDT.

Something else useful to know- for a lot of us, it took months to years of tinkering to dial in our optimal dose. You also need an awareness that if you gain or lose weight, or other health factors change, you might need a shift in medication doses. Stay with it until it's right and plan on having an active and ongoing conversation with your medical team on your supplemental thyroid dosing.

OH! We were also recently shocked to discover some doctors were neglecting to tell their patients that *they must take their thyroid meds on an empty stomach (usually upon waking), and refrain from eating or drinking for 60 minutes post-ingestion.* We thought we'd better let you know you need to do that or you won't absorb all the meds!

Did you know that a dysregulated thyroid can affect your cholesterol numbers?
Because the thyroid is a major player in energy utilization, it makes sense that it can impact your lipids readings. If you have ongoing issues with your lipid readings, it can be a clue that your thyroid is possibly out of whack (that's the technical term).

THYROID NOTES: Nutrients

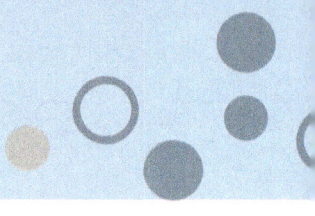

Thyroid hormones are very sensitive to nutrient intake - truly one of the most basic ways to tank your thyroid hormones is plain old under-eating- there are also a few specific nutrients that are especially important to our thyroid function.

* Iodine * Selenium * L-Tyrosine * Iron *Vitamin A * Zinc * Copper *

Proper iodine intake is essential to thyroid health. Even if you use "iodized" (aka with added iodine) salt, you possibly aren't getting what you need and a lot of us who are focused on healthy eating use "cleaner" salt that doesn't add supplemental iodine. That doesn't mean you have to go back to the Umbrella Girl version -it simply means you need to make sure to get it from other sources.

(Note: in health circles, there is some discussion of hyper-supplementation of iodine, at much higher than RDA levels. We are not recommending that here. We simply want to make sure you are getting the effective dose.)

Iodine combines with L-Tyrosine (an amino acid made from another amino acid, phenylalanine) assisted by Selenium to create thyroid hormone.

The great news is that the remaining nutrients of concern: Iron, Vitamin A, Zinc, and Copper as well as Selenium and L-Tyrosine precursors are all found easily in food. If your diet is based on high-quality animal-based protein sources like shellfish, fish, beef, pork, chicken, eggs, some aged cheeses, a bit of liver, seeds, and some leafy greens, you should get sufficient quantities of these nutrients.

Seaweed is a great source of iodine, as are fish and shellfish. If you are not a fish or seaweed consumer, you may look at iodine supplementation.

Vegetarians and Vegans are the populations at the highest risk for low selenium as well as most of these other essential nutrients and will need to look at supplementing.

A NOTE ABOUT BRAZIL NUTS

Brazil Nuts are often cited as a great source of selenium. They are indeed incredibly high in nutrients! A single brazil nut delivers well over the daily RDA. The upper safe limit of daily selenium is 400 mg - so exceeding 4-5 nuts per day can lead to selenium toxicity - which should be avoided! So a few is fine, a lot is not. But if you eat sufficient quantities of meat, you get plenty without adding brazil nuts to your diet.

WHAT IS A GOITER?

Goiters used to be much more common, but you seldom see them these days.

In the 1920's the US began adding iodine to salt, to help correct the common problem, as iodine deficiency was then understood to be a cause of goiter. Interestingly this iodine supplementation of salt actually raised the average IQ in the United States. This is because iodine is crucial for cognitive development and function. (GO IODINE!)

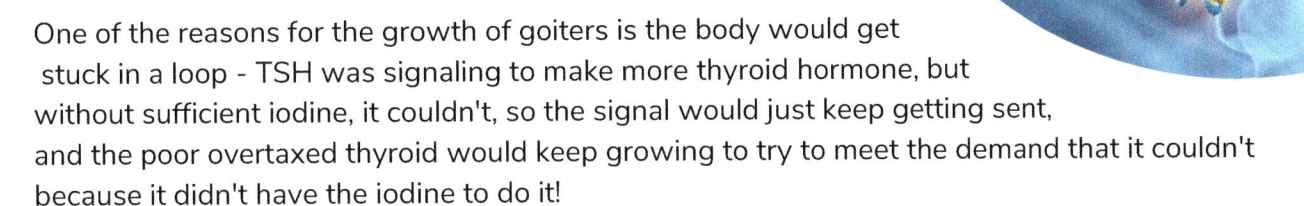

One of the reasons for the growth of goiters is the body would get stuck in a loop - TSH was signaling to make more thyroid hormone, but without sufficient iodine, it couldn't, so the signal would just keep getting sent, and the poor overtaxed thyroid would keep growing to try to meet the demand that it couldn't because it didn't have the iodine to do it!

What people might not realize is thyroid nodules, which we still do see today, are smaller versions. A goiter is simply a thyroid nodule that grows to the point it is visible externally.

Low iodine was not the only cause of goiter, simply the most common. Hyperthyroid, hypothyroid and autoimmune thyroiditis can also cause nodules and goiters.
Some types of nodules need to be biopsied as there is a small chance of cancer.

If you have any swelling in the region of the thyroid, be sure get that checked out! Iodine deficiency can be easily treated, however if it's something more serious, you don't want to delay treatment.

One last note on Thyroid:

If you are already on Thyroid Medication, consult with your doctor about dosing on the day of the blood draw. Most doctors will have you delay your dose from the morning of the blood draw until after the blood is drawn. However, some doctors have different protocols, and the timing of meds will affect the interpretation of results. So make sure you are on the same page!

SEX HORMONE BASICS

Again and again, we hear from folks who hit their 40's and 50's and feel run down and tired. When they finally ask their doctor about it, they are brushed off. "What do you expect? You aren't young anymore!"

We've already hit on the thyroid as an area of inquiry when you feel off, but we need to talk about another one, especially if your 30's are in your rearview mirror. Sex Hormones. While hormone dysfunction can strike at any age, our sex hormones become a specific area of greater concern as we enter our middle years. Although, for some of us, dysfunction can happen sooner, especially when someone suffers from metabolic illnesses.

We felt this was something we needed to discuss as proper hormone levels are crucial to feeling well! Some doctors have discouraged testing of sex hormones because they won't support intervening with hormone therapy, so they'd say "why bother testing?" They won't support supplementing hormones because they have been swayed by poorly run (or badly interpreted) studies, while others hold outdated belief systems that keep them from helping their patients live optimal lives.
They'll often say things like, "Menopause is normal. It's just something you have to deal with."

Hot flashes. Reduced Bladder Control. Mood Swings. Poor Sleep. Weight Gain. Muscles Loss. Loss of Sex Drive. Painful Sex. Acne. Depression. Bone Loss. Thinning hair. Painful Joints... do these sound like things that should just be put up with as part of normal aging if there is treatment that can improve your life experience?

Menopause in women, and Andropause in men are age related declines in sex hormones. When these lead to feeling run down and less optimal we strongly support hormone supplementation with Bio-Identical Hormone therapy. Some people (especially metabolically healthy ones) zip through this hormonal change without feeling bad at all, but if you do suffer from symptoms there should be no shame or hesitation to correct those declining hormones.

We understand if your doctor is not on board with treating your symptoms, that can be a really frustrating situation. Unfortunately, sometimes you have to seek out new practitioners when your current one stops being in alignment with being a supportive health partner.

Time of Day Matters: Sex Hormones can shift through the day, so time of day matters!
The same person might show a total Testosterone of 500 in the morning but only 375 later that same day! Make sure you aren't mistaking timing issues for Hormone issues! Also, some seasonal variation has been noted.

In this book, we will give you the specific hormones you want to assess if you are still in functional ranges. We'll break this down into male and female specific labs. The tests we mention here give a really great baseline check-in. Additional follow-up hormone tests not listed here may be required should an imbalance be discovered.

FEMALE SPECIFIC SEX HORMONES (RECOMMENDED TESTS)

Estradiol is a specific type of estrogen produced in the ovaries. This is a central marker of female hormone production, and what is typically evaluated in labs. The level expected in the blood is cycle timing-dependent.
Progesterone is a hormone that rises in the second half of a menstruating woman's cycle, but it is always present and needed at all times at an appropriate level.
Sex hormone-binding globulin (SHBG) is a liver protein that binds to sex hormones for distribution. When hormones are bound, they are unavailable. All hormones are either in bound or free versions. We need to know how much of our hormones are free, as that is the version available to use.
Total Testosterone is traditionally thought of as a male sex hormone however, it is also necessary in females. Yes, women need testosterone! Especially if they want to feel good, sleep well, maintain good body composition, and have a sex drive.

MALE SPECIFIC SEX HORMONES (RECOMMENDED TESTS)

Total Testosterone is a traditionally male sex hormone that helps men develop androgenic (traditionally male) features and enhances sex drive and muscular development. Total Testosterone refers to the combination of free and bound forms, so the total amount.
Free Testosterone is testosterone not bound up with other proteins and is free for use in the blood.
Zinc is a vitamin that is essential for the body to properly use testosterone. So low zinc levels might be implicated in poor testosterone.
Sex hormone-binding globulin (SHBG) is a liver protein that binds to sex hormones for distribution.
For men over 50, we also recommend testing:
PSA (Prostate-Specific Androgen) test.
This can help monitor prostate issues on the (hopefully distant) horizon.

THE PARATHYROID

What is the difference between the parathyroid and the thyroid?

A Parathyroid gland actually has nothing to do with the Thyroid other than being neighbors. The parathyroid is simply located on the back of the thyroid, hence the prefix: para, which means near. There are 4 Parathyroid glands, and their job is to regulate the calcium and phosphorus levels in the body.

The symptoms associated with parathyroid issues are often shrugged off as "aging," but if the Parathyroid gland is not functioning right, you need to rule out active parathyroid cancer, and confirm that it is merely hyperparathyroidism.
However, even this "benign" form of dysregulation increases the risk of many types of cancer, heart issues, and other medical conditions. It can decrease life expectancy and life enjoyment, so it should be managed and monitored.

Symptoms of a outta-whack Parathyroid commonly include: Chronic Fatigue, Depressed Mood, Bone and/or Muscle pain, nausea or abdominal pain, constipation, frequent urination, mental fogginess, heart palpitations, kidney stones, slow thinking/cognition, heartburn, osteopenia, or osteoporosis.

Parathyroid dysregulation is so frequently missed that we felt it important to bring it up in this book. This is one reason why it's so important to check a calcium level. So...

If the Serum Calcium level is elevated at all, even off by .1, you should be getting all of these follow-up tests:

- **Intact PTH**
- **Ionized Calcium**
- **Phosphorus**
- **Fractionated Alkaline Phosphatase**
- **Vitamin D -25**

If any of the first four listed come back abnormal, you should get an ultrasound or CAT Scan of the Parathyroid glands. Vitamin D-25 can be off for a variety of unrelated reasons.

JENNIFER'S PARATHYROID

Jennifer is a mom of two teenagers who had just turned 55, and at her physical she complained of feeling run down and exhausted. She struggled to keep up with her busy job as a vet tech.

"Just part of getting older," her doctor assured her. "There's nothing of concern on your labs."

If he'd checked her calcium levels, he'd have found them just above normal. A lot of doctors might not pick up on the fact that anything out of range on calcium should be considered a big red flag, so they don't follow up on it.

Several months passed, with Jennifer feeling increasingly low. Tired, run-down, no energy - she was told to exercise more because being out of shape made her tired. And while it's true regular exercise can help energy levels, she didn't even have enough energy to try to move more. She just wanted to nap all the time.

When the tiredness progressed to rapid weight loss, her doctor initially thought that was great, until she explained it wasn't from her increased exercise, as she was now barely able to leave the couch and had to take leave from her job. That's when he finally ran some additional labs. Her calcium was now elevated by several points - a condition known as Hypercalcemia - which is very dangerous.

More advanced testing revealed the cause of her high calcium was a parathyroid tumor. Once removed, her calcium levels returned to normal and she felt so much better!

It's so easy to dismiss symptoms of true issues as, "Just getting older, I guess." Feeling terrible is NOT a sign of normal aging. Don't let anyone try to tell you it is.

COMMON SENSE LABS DIAGNOSES OF EXCLUSION

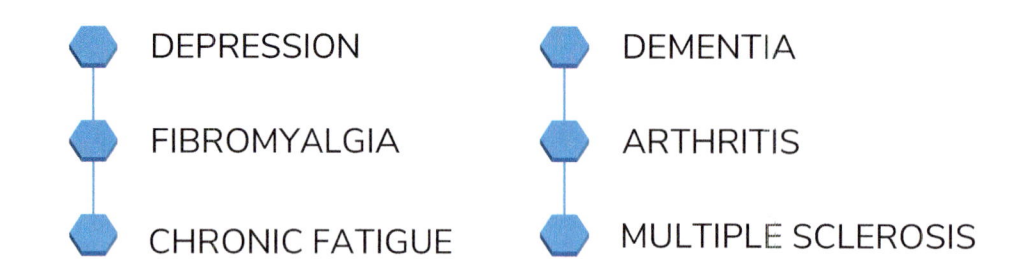

- DEPRESSION
- FIBROMYALGIA
- CHRONIC FATIGUE
- DEMENTIA
- ARTHRITIS
- MULTIPLE SCLEROSIS

There are several conditions that should not be diagnosed solely by discussion of symptoms, or from a single lab marker, but often are diagnosed in exactly this way by many doctors.
These are called diagnoses of exclusion because your doctor must run comprehensive lab tests to **exclude** other similar issues.

You or someone you love may have been diagnosed with one of these, or similar conditions; it is imperative that you understand how they **should** be diagnosed. In this case a misdiagnosis will almost inevitably result in mistreatment.

Misdiagnosis are more likely happen in our overburdened medical climate when doctors aren't given the time they'd need for a complex diagnosis. These diseases don't have a simple test that proves the diagnosis, rather they are a list of symptoms, many of which might also reflect other conditions. You need to rule out a multitude of other diagnoses presenting with similar symptoms before you can diagnose the above conditions with any degree of accuracy. However, we see significant numbers of folks coming into the clinic on medications to treat an illness, and upon further investigation, we find that they do not actually have that illness - so the meds they were given are at best, ineffective, and at worst, health and wellness damaging.

Misdiagnosis means you may suffer for years, decades, or even your whole life because you aren't getting the treatment that would actually help the condition from which you suffer. On top of that, you might be pharmaceutically treated for a totally different condition - one you may not have. A medical double whammy of harm.

KIM'S MISDIAGNOSIS

When I was in elementary school, I suffered a serious bout of depression. Daily tears, thoughts of worthlessness, and a lack of drive or desire to do anything. At that time, I was put in therapy, with no medical check-in to see if my symptoms might be related to anything hormonal.

I spent the next several years fluctuating between sort of ok and extremely not ok, but then more symptoms began to appear, most notably hair loss, exhaustion, and being cold most of the time. I could function. I could get through my days, I even had good days where I was happy and felt ok, but they were not most days.

This functional, yet not optimal, situation persisted for the next decade and a half before I had a few months where things got worse. At that time I was escalated to a visit with a psychiatrist to prescribe medication: Anti-depressants. When those had no effect (well, beyond rapid weight gain) they decided I must be bipolar, and they put me on bipolar meds - which also did nothing to help.

After I had had enough of taking pills that didn't help and tapered off and just went about my life, assuming that was the best I could do.

Fast forward to decades later when I was diagnosed with hypothyroidism. As I was going over my history with my doctor, she said, "I'd bet good money you've been dealing with this since you were a pre-teen." Light bulb moment.

From Dr. Berry, I've learned that my depression as a child was improperly diagnosed. Depression should be seen as a diagnosis of exclusion; running many tests to rule out alternative health issues. They weren't. As a child, I was lucky to have health insurance, so It wasn't due to a lack of resources that I wasn't properly tested, it was a lack of thorough evaluation from the doctor. Even in the best scenario, with comprehensive medical insurance, I got under-treated. With the state of medical care now, I imagine it's worse for so many people.

From that point on, since I already had depression in my chart when I had worsening symptoms, they automatically assumed it was related to that depression - so I was pigeonholed into treatment options, rather than anyone taking a good look at the root causes and if a different diagnosis was a better fit.

Section 4:
Blood Glucose Monitoring

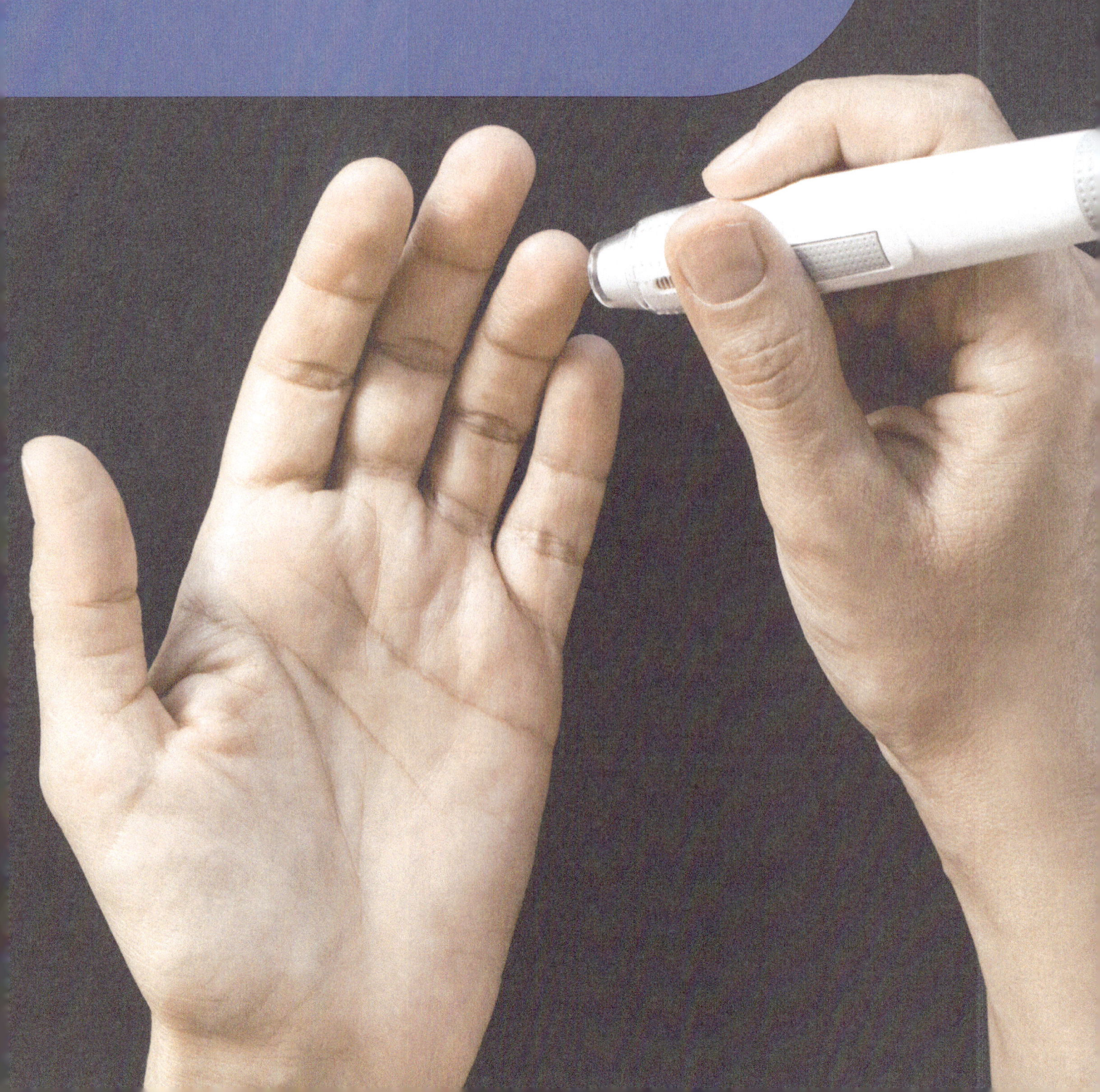

SPECIAL SECTION: BLOOD GLUCOSE MONITORING

Some lab tests, such as glucose, get checked in the lab panels, but this is an isolated single reading that might not provide enough information to be useful due to its high variability. There are some options for at-home monitoring, so we thought we'd discuss a few of the most common (and possibly beneficial) ones. We'd love it if there were more available- like Insulin! - but for now, these are what is available and we see can be of benefit to some folks.

We are huge proponents of tracking blood sugar (another way to say blood glucose, often shortened to BG). Our body's ability to keep glucose in a healthy range is so important to long-term health. In a healthy person, the body is brilliant at maintaining glucose homeostasis - the body seeks balance in all things, including glucose in our blood. We are brilliantly created to have a glucose regulation system housed in our pancreas. Is your blood sugar too low? Glucagon signals the release of more glucose. Too high? Insulin signals the storage of glucose and turns down the release of your body's store of glycogen (the name for stored glucose). Amazing!

Unfortunately, as many of you are aware when we become insulin resistant, these systems can break down and we lose our tendency to naturally achieve balance. This can lead to wildly swinging blood sugar levels.

By monitoring your blood glucose, you can get real-time feedback that you are eating in a way that will help your body improve glucose management. Rather than being prey to the swings of blood sugar, you can "eat to your meter" and keep your blood sugar in healthy ranges. Over time, this can lead to major health improvements.

In a person that has lost good internal glucose management due to insulin resistance, actively physically monitoring glucose at home becomes imperative to healing and long-term health.

You might think, "Isn't monitoring A1c and fasting glucose enough?" Unfortunately, not always. A1c only gives us a proxy for our average blood sugar, and that's only part of the picture. If your blood sugar is sometimes low and other times very high, your average will look fine, but your body is suffering from the high variability and the frequent high blood sugar excursions are causing damage.

Glucose Homeostasis

The automatic balance of insulin & glucagon to maintain steady blood sugars.

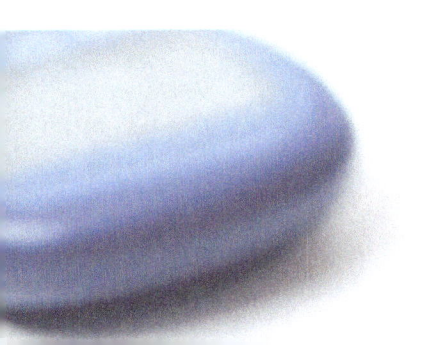

GLUCOSE MONITORING METHODS

There are two methods to monitor your glucose at home.
The most accessible is the glucometer - no prescription is required and they are relatively low cost. These can be affordably purchased in most pharmacies or online. Often colloquially referred to as "finger-prick testing" - you simply poke your (clean!) finger with a lancet, which allows a small drop of blood to surface, and apply that blood to a test strip inserted into the glucometer, which will give you a reading of your approximate* blood glucose at that time. This method is easy to get, and while not complicated to use, can be a bit tedious as every measurement requires a finger prick and test strip.

The second method is using a Continuous Glucose Monitor (CGM). In the United States, CGMs require a prescription and are more costly than a glucometer. (Although more direct-to-consumer services such as Nutrisense and Levels are popping up every day.)
This consists of a little sticky sensor pad that is applied to your arm (or stomach for some models) and has a small filament that measures your interstitial fluid (just under the skin) which tracks pretty closely with your blood glucose. The sensor wirelessly transmits the readings to an app where you can see the readout.

Each of these methods (glucometer or CGM) has pluses and minuses.
The CGM is ever-ready and you can get multiple readings across a day without constantly having to prick your finger. But it requires a prescription (or use of a service), not to mention the increased cost. Also, something to be aware of - since it's testing a slightly different fluid, there can be a 10-15 minute delay on changes in readings. Additionally, we find absolute numbers on a CGM to be slightly less accurate than glucometers. Questionable readings always need cross-checking with a glucometer to confirm them.
Because the glucometer is a bit more of a hassle to use, this sometimes leads to incomplete monitoring as you don't always want to stop what you are doing, clean your finger, open a test strip, prick your finger, test the blood, again and again over a day.

Accuracy

We can't emphasize enough that blood sugar monitoring either with CGM or glucometer has a fairly high margin for error of 20%. While we find the glucometer slightly more trustworthy in terms of accuracy, it is still not sensitive enough to interpret small changes.

We constantly see folks trying to figure out the reason this reading was 89, but this other reading was 94... truth is, based on the sensitivity of the meter, those readings are basically the same. If this imprecision will drive you crazy - perhaps monitoring is not for you.

59

TARGETED BLOOD SUGAR RANGES

As we mentioned, A1c is not enough for everyone to confirm they are in good glucose control. While A1c can somewhat stand in for one of the things you want to track, average glucose, it leaves out two other important considerations:

1. Fasting & Between Meal Glucose levels: BG in the "unfed" state.
2. MAGE (Mean Amplitude of Glycemic Excursions) or BG variability over the day.

In simple terms, you want your blood sugar to do this: Your baseline glucose levels start the day in a healthy range, then should not go too high due to what you eat, and then should come back to that healthy baseline relatively quickly after your meal. Makes sense, doesn't it?

So, what should the glucose range be after overnight fasting or between meals?

There's a bit of individual variability, but we believe in most cases, numbers should fall in these ranges when out of the post-prandial (after meal) window.

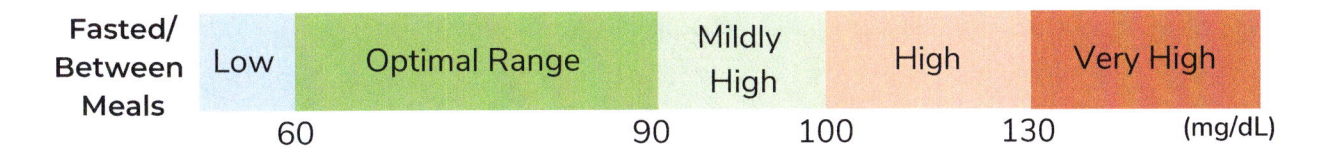

Fasted/Between Meals	Low	Optimal Range	Mildly High	High	Very High
	60	90	100	130	(mg/dL)

These ranges are quite different than those you see recommended by organizations such as the American Diabetes Association (ADA). However, as we have seen time and time again, cut-off points for many readings are way too high for true good health. Here we are presenting you with what we believe to be best based on Dr. Berry's clinical experience and also studies on achieving optimal outcomes.

Additionally, we don't give different targets for diabetics vs non-diabetics, as the ADA does. While we understand diabetics will struggle more to keep glucose in optimal ranges, that doesn't mean we should lie to them about what is optimal. Rome wasn't built in a day, and a diabetic won't fix their numbers overnight either, however, they can set their GPS on the right target and make steps towards their desired destination daily. Direction matters more than speed!

OUTLIERS & EXCEPTIONS

There are some circumstances when your numbers might fall out of these ranges without it being an area of concern. Here are a few of the most common examples:

Keto and/or Multiday Fasting: Some people might experience a fasting glucose in the "low" range, falling in the 50s, and in the proper circumstances (paired with appropriately high Ketones) is not usually a concern as long as they are feeling and functioning well.

Dawn Phenomenon: Some folks notice an early morning peak in glucose. This is a short rise in glucose right after waking due to naturally higher cortisol production. Dawn Phenomenon is a normal physiological process and occurs in every mammal on Earth, to some degree. Don't stress too much if there's a transient reading just after waking, as long as it's under approximately 125, and readings at other times are all in the right range. Because of Dawn Phenomenon, we recommend testing "fasting" blood glucose once you've been up and about for an hour or two rather than right after hopping out of bed.

Exercise: Vigorous movement can temporarily raise glucose in a short window, but over time, exercise lowers average glucose levels, so it's a benefit on the whole. Don't freak out if your glucose goes into the high range for a short period of time during and/or right after a workout.

Hot or Cold: Submersion in very hot or very cold water can raise or lower glucose temporarily. This can be due to a variety of reasons such as changes in cortisol or blood flow.

Average Blood Glucose

As mentioned in the description of A1c, most doctors will use A1c as a proxy measure (surrogate marker) for average blood glucose over the last 90 days. While we certainly think tracking A1c is a useful measurement for most folks, (barring genetic variants that make it a less accurate measure) there's a benefit to instead tracking average glucose over a shorter time frame, especially if trying to implement changes.

If using a CGM, finding your average glucose is as easy as looking at the reports section of your app. If you are tracking through a glucometer, you'd need to be getting regular readings each day to have enough data to pull from to determine accurate average blood sugar and see the trends and patterns of your blood sugar levels.

Note: Average Glucose is over 24-hour daily cycles, so will include both fed and fasted periods.

79		100	108		114	mg/dL
	Optimal Range		OK	Slightly High	High	
4.4		5.1	5.4		5.6	a1C %

Above we've shown the average glucose as well as the corresponding A1c level. Maintaining anything under 108 mg/dl (5.4% A1c) average glucose keeps you in the range that avoids most damage from chronic high blood sugars, but keeping things under 100 mg/dL seems to have a slight health advantage.

While the ADA doesn't call it pre-diabetes until your average glucose reaches 118 mg/dL (5.7% A1c), we think this is too high a limit marker. When the average glucose rises above 108 mg/dl (5.4% A1c), we begin to see damage from occasional high blood sugars.
Obviously, the damage increases exponentially the higher these numbers go.

MAGE: Mean Amplitude of Glucose Excursions

MAGE (Mean Amplitude of Glycemic Excursions) is an average of how much glucose levels fluctuate. This is important because you might have two people who both maintain an average blood glucose of 95 mg/dl.
But person A has **high** variability with glucose going as high as 150 mg/dl at times, and as low as 70mg/dl at others. Person B has **low** variability, with their glucose always staying within 85 to 105 mg/dl. The health of these people may well be very different, as higher variability indicates poorer health outcomes.

Things that are known to cause Glycemic Excursions (which some call "Spikes" - an excursion is the period of time glucose remains elevated from baseline):

- Stress. Some people report their highest blood sugar of the day is on their commute or after an argument.

- Dehydration. This one is not actually raising your absolute glucose, but rather increasing the concentration of sugar in the blodo, as the blood volume decreased due to lack of water.

- Eating or drinking, especially high-carbohydrate foods and beverages. Alcohol can actually drop blood glucose - in fact, alcoholics often have very low average glucose. In this case, low blood sugar is not a good thing as it is caused by subversion of normal liver processes.

For most people, perhaps unsurprisingly, but importantly, the main cause of blood sugar variability is in their food choices. Which makes testing specifically before and after eating an especially useful practice to help avoid large glucose excursions.

Prandial: during or related to the eating of food.

Terms frequently used in discussing blood sugars are preprandial and postprandial. Preprandial refers to the time before a meal, and postprandial refers to the period after a meal.

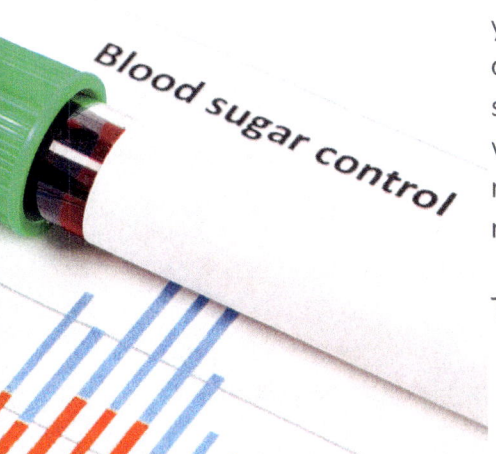

When monitoring pre and postprandial glucose, you can learn your degree of carb tolerance. You might also learn that glycemic control is about specific food choices rather than simply a carb or sugar amount. Hummus might spike your blood sugars super high, while bananas do nothing or vice versa. By testing your glucose response to foods, there can be a benefit to learning your unique response as there can be a high degree of personal variability.

There are two important factors in terms of Postprandial numbers:
1. How high the Blood Glucose goes.
2. How long Blood Glucose stays elevated.

POSTPRANDIAL BLOOD SUGAR

Postprandial glucose management is the practice of monitoring your glucose levels after you've eaten a meal. The degree of rise, in relationship to the pre-meal number, is an indication of your level of insulin resistance. Note your glucose reading immediately before eating, record its highest point, then monitor how long it takes to return to baseline. Compare those figures to the chart below to determine if you're in the "great" or "needs improvement" range.

How High?

The first factor we mentioned in postprandial number management is watching where excursion peaked. Our recommendation is that your post meal BG reading should be no more than **30 points** (in mg/dl) higher than the preprandial number. (Don't forget to include there's a margin of error in all readings.)

We are giving you optimal ranges here. Please do not expect perfection on day one. Small incremental improvements will add up. Use the optimal numbers as a point to aim towards, not a reason to beat yourself up. Developing good blood sugar control can take some time. For example, when Kim first went on Keto, she'd regularly see her blood sugar go up 40-50 points after a meal. A year later the exact same meals would only cause a 10-20 point elevation. These optimal ranges are your target to aim towards. Just keep heading in the right direction, and trust you'll get there.

For How Long?

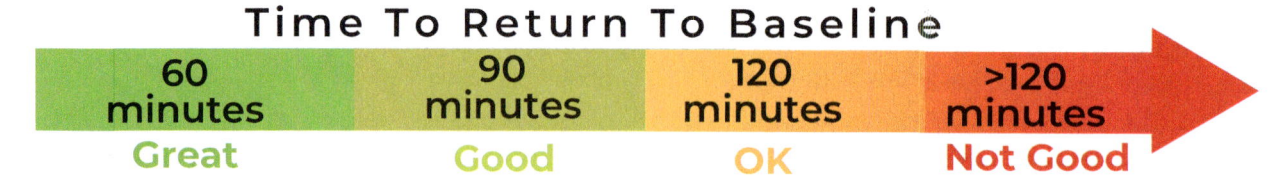

Time To Return To Baseline

60 minutes	90 minutes	120 minutes	>120 minutes
Great	Good	OK	Not Good

The two primary things to manipulate if your numbers aren't to your liking:

1. The composition of your meal. What types of foods you choose to eat will have the biggest affect on glucose level. Carbohydrates have the greatest impact on glucose levels.
2. The size of your meal. A large meal will often have more of an affect than a small one.

While not all blood sugar issues can be managed solely through diet, food choices always play a central role in any long-term management strategy.

Important Note: If you have been eating very low carbs and then suddenly have a high-carb food, your blood glucose will overreact due to insufficient insulin readiness. Do not panic, this is a temporary insufficiency due to the downregulation of insulin production. If you are metabolically healthy and ate higher carbs for a few days, your insulin production would return to a level better able to handle the higher carbohydrate load. Not that we are suggesting it - just something of which to be aware!

A TALE OF TWO DIETS

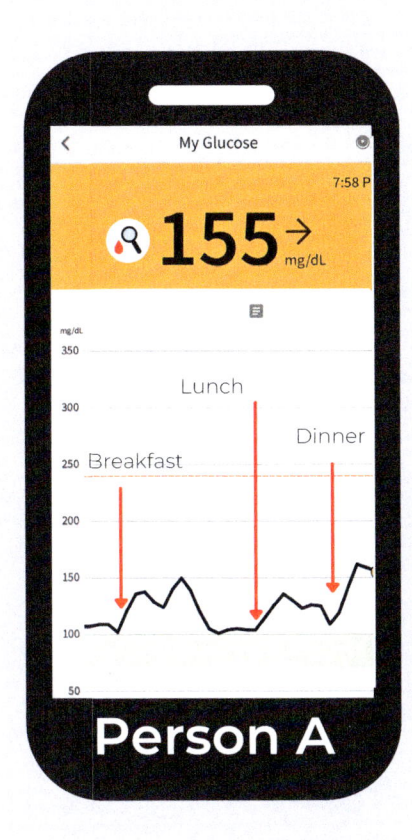

Person A's glucose before breakfast was hovering just over 100, so slightly high for a fasting BG, then after eating breakfast we see their glucose rise to 150, well above the desired maximum rise of 30 points. Also, note there's a double peak after breakfast - that can happen when the body is fighting hard to bring the glucose down, but their insulin response gets overwhelmed, and a second rise happens right away. You also see how long glucose remained elevated.

Then after lunch, we see a rise of about 40 points, and right as the glucose began to drop, it was dinner time, and boom, blood sugar went back up a good 50 points.
You see that Person A spent very little time in their day at lower blood sugar levels and in fact, spent the whole day over "optimal" levels.

Person A might not be diagnosed as diabetic by the mainstream medical system, but we can tell you that if someone's glucose looked like this most days, we'd be concerned about them.

Person B's morning glucose was about 75, and after breakfast, it only rose a very small amount, maybe 5 points, and the same at lunch. The rises from her breakfast and lunch were so minor they are indistinguishable from natural variations without food.

There was a more definitive rise after dinner, about 15-20 points that then dripped back to the pre-meal level very quickly.

Does someone have to be this flatlined to be healthy? No, some rise and fall are fine and natural, but there are many folks who find their glucose levels with very little fluctuations- especially when on a low carbohydrate diet.

While young, you might not see significant health differences between Person A and B, but over time, there would be a widening health gap, with Person A seeing a growing level of health deterioration.

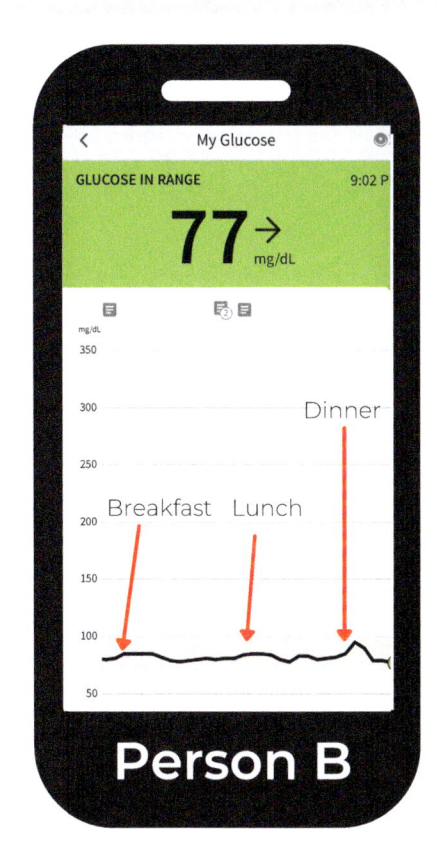

SHOULD EVERYONE TRACK?

Some Common Sense Advice:
Ultimately, not everyone will find self-monitoring of blood sugar useful. If you are active and metabolically healthy, with no history of blood sugar dysregulation, it's unlikely you need to monitor your blood sugar. However, we see no problem with someone like this wanting to appease a curiosity and see how your body responds to certain foods by monitoring for a short time.

We believe blood sugar monitoring to have to most beneficial for folks who are not seeing the type of glycemic control they think they should be based on their diet.
For instance, if someone doesn't understand why their A1C is higher than they think it should be, or they eat a mixed diet and aren't sure if that's ok for their body or not, a period of self-exploration can be very useful!

Do I need to track forever?

Some folks freak out over the idea that once they start to track their glucose they'll need to do so forever. Don't fret about that one, it's not true. We are creatures of habit. We tend to eat the same thing over and over. So, if you track for 2 weeks or a month and see your body is responding well to your chosen foods, you can stop and rest easy in the knowledge that the trend of good responses should continue.
If you find your body responding unfavorably to your choices, we'd continue tracking until you dial in the best options for your glucose ranges.

WHO SHOULD BE CAUTIOUS?

We want to bring up two issues we repeated see with glucose self-monitoring:

OVER-THINKING: As we mentioned earlier, there's a limit to the precision and accuracy of these meters (and all testing!) So if you are going to fixate on why your glucose went from 85 to 90 when you ate or drank that thing... stop and evaluate your expectations. If the imprecision of the meter is going to eat at you, you might be causing yourself INCREASED harm by stressing over things that are out of your hands and actually don't really exist, to begin with. You can not make meaning out of changes under the limit of the accuracy of your tools. Many folks try, but they are just spinning in the land of imagination. Keep to reality for sanity's sake.

MISTAKEN PRIORITIES: We sometimes see people getting upset about any rise in glucose, mistakenly thinking that a completely flat line on their CGM is the goal. In this case, we sometimes see people making poor nutritional decisions (not eating enough protein, nutrient deficiencies, etc) in pursuit of this. While we don't want big spikes, some postprandial excursions - within tolerance ranges (see page 60-63) are perfectly healthy.

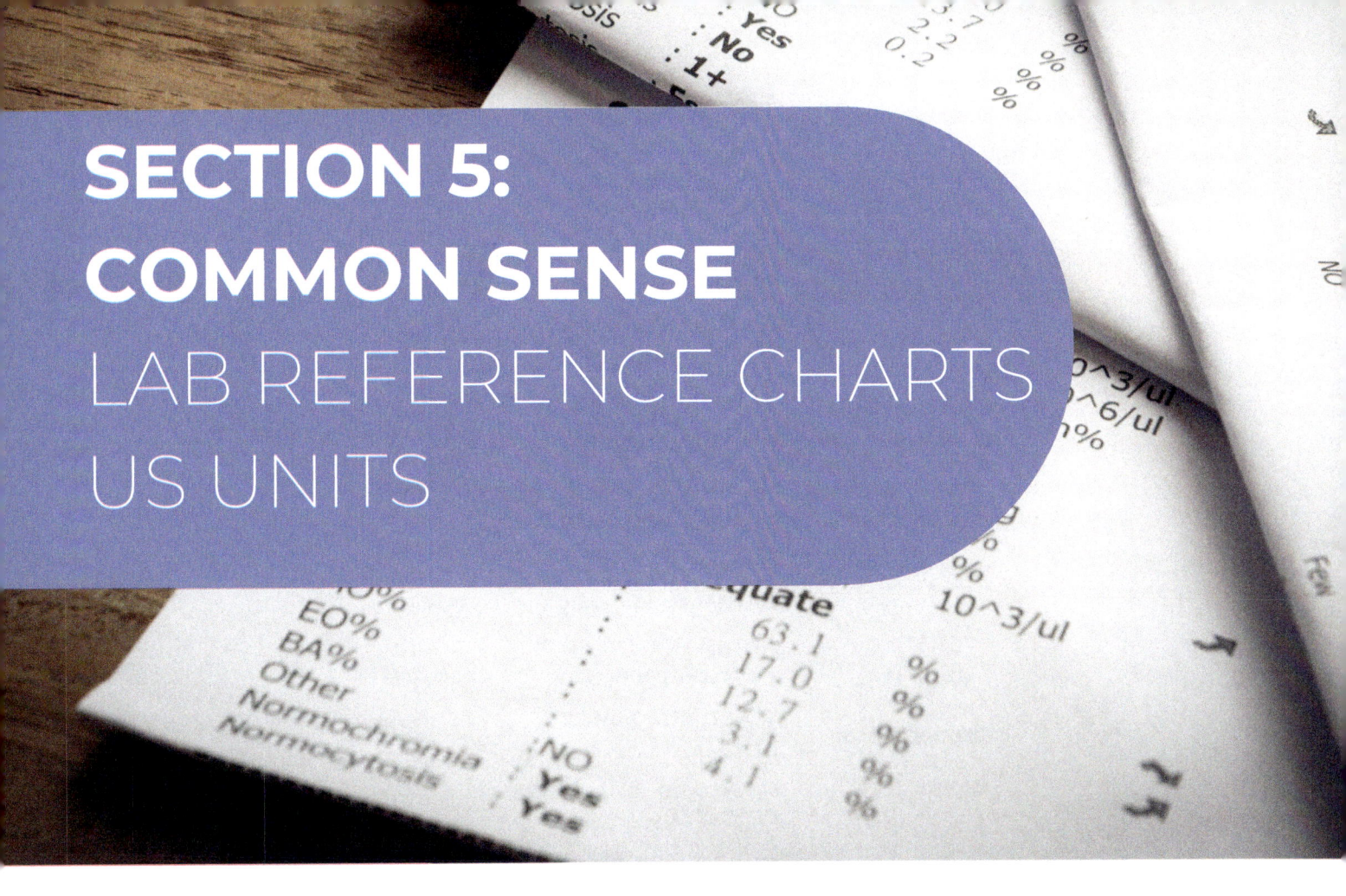

SECTION 5: COMMON SENSE LAB REFERENCE CHARTS US UNITS

The information provided within the following charts is for informational and educational purposes only.

Please consult a trusted healthcare professional before making any medication or health decisions. These ranges are not designed to diagnose, treat, or cure any disease. Acceptance of these ranges varies based on practitioner.

We primarily use US based units in this book as the authors are US based. However, at the end of this section you'll find SI units for our friends in other nations!

A few things you'll want to note: some labs, even within the same country, will note things differently. So always check the units to make sure you are comparing apples to apples!

Annual Labs: CMP

A Comprehensive Metabolic Panel reflects blood levels of proteins & electrolytes & glucose levels. These tests reflect the health of your liver, kidneys, bones, muscle cells, nerve and cell function.

TEST/PANEL	LABS	RANGE	UNITS	PERSONAL DATA
CMP	Albumin	STANDARD 3.50-5.50 OPTIMAL 4.0-5.0	g/dL	
	Albumin/Globulin Ratio	STANDARD 1.20-2.20 OPTIMAL 1.40-2.10	Ratio	
	Alkaline Phosphotase	STANDARD 39.0-117.0 OPTIMAL 70.0-100.0	IU/L	
	ALT (SGOT)	STANDARD 0.0-44.0 OPTIMAL 10.0-26.0	IU/L	
	AST (SGPT)	STANDARD 0.0-40.0 OPTIMAL 10.0-26.0	IU/L	
	Biliruben Total	STANDARD 0.0-1.20 OPTIMAL 0.10-0.90	mg/dL	
	Blood Urea Nitrogen (BUN)*	STANDARD 6.0 - 24.0 OPTIMAL 10.0 - 20.0	mg/dL	
	BUN/Creatinine*	STANDARD 9.0-20.0 OPTIMAL 10.0-20.0	Ratio	
	Calcium	STANDARD 8.70-10.20 OPTIMAL 9.20-10.0	mg/dL	
	Carbon Dioxide	STANDARD 20.0-29.0 OPTIMAL 25.0-29.0	MEq/L	
	Creatinine*	STANDARD 0.76-1.27 OPTIMAL 0.70 - 1.10	mg/dL	
	Globulin, total	STANDARD 1.50-4.50 OPTIMAL 2.40 - 2.80	g/dL	
	Glucose (Fasting)	STANDARD 65.0-99.0 OPTIMAL 65.0 - 86.0	mg/dL	
	Potassium	STANDARD 3.50-5.20 OPTIMAL 4.00 - 4.50	MEq/L	
	Protein, total	STANDARD 6.0-8.50 OPTIMAL 6.90 - 7.40	g/dL	
	Sodium	STANDARD 134.0-144.0 OPTIMAL 134.0-144.0	MEq/L	
	Sodium to Potassium Ratio	STANDARD 30.0-35.0 OPTIMAL 30.0-35.0	Ratio	

*Creatinine and BUN levels may be elevated if you have high muscle mass or have eaten red meat in the last 24 hours. Higher serum levels than listed due to these reasons are not problematic.

Cystatin C is a blood marker that can be alternatively tested that will show kidney function more clearly in these cases.

Annual Labs: CBC

The CBC looks at levels of components of White and Red Blood cells to evaluate Infections. Allergic Reactions, Blood Volume, Oxygenation, blood clotting and Immune functions.

TEST	LABS	RANGE	UNITS	PERSONAL DATA
COMPLETE BLOOD COUNT (CBC) W DIFF *Reminder to check units. Labcorp writes these "absolute" values in x10E3/uL while Quest lab lists them as cells/uL meaning the decimal place will very different depending on the lab you visited Easy conversion, just a reminder to pay attention to units	Baso (Absolute)*	STANDARD 0.0 - 0.2 OPTIMAL 0.0 - 0.2	x10E3/uL	
	Basos	NOT ESTABLISHED	%	
	EOS	NOT ESTABLISHED	%	
	EOS (Absolute)*	STANDARD 0.0 - 0.4 OPTIMAL 0.0 - 0.4	x10E3/uL	
	Hematocrit	STANDARD 34 -36.6 OPTIMAL 34 - 36.6	%	
	Hemoglobin	STANDARD 11.1 - 15.9 OPTIMAL 11.1 - 15.9	g/dL	
	Immature Grans (Absolute)*	STANDARD 0.0 - 0.1 OPTIMAL 0.0 - 0.1	x10E3/uL	
	Immature Granulocytes	NOT ESTABLISHED	%	
	Lymphs	NOT ESTABLISHED	%	
	Lymphs (Absolute)*	STANDARD 0.7 -3.1 OPTIMAL 0.7 -3.1	x10E3/uL	
	MCH	STANDARD 26.6 - 33.0 OPTIMAL 26.6 - 33.0	pg	
	MCV	STANDARD 79 -97 OPTIMAL 79 - 97	fL	
	Monocytes	NOT ESTABLISHED	%	
	Monocytes (Absolute)*	STANDARD 0.1 - 0.9 OPTIMAL 0.1 - 0.9	x10E3/uL	
	Neutrophils	NOT ESTABLISHED	%	
	Neutrophils (Absolute)*	STANDARD 1.4 - 7.0 OPTIMAL 1.4 - 7.0	x10E3/uL	
	Platelets	STANDARD 150-379 OPTIMAL 150 - 379	%	
	RDW	STANDARD 12.3- 15.4 OPTIMAL 12.3 - 15.4	x10E3/uL	
	Red Blood Cells (RBC)	STANDARD 3.77 - 5.28 OPTIMAL 3.77 - 5.28	x10E3/uL	
	White Blood Cells (WBC)	STANDARD 3.4 - 10.8 OPTIMAL 3.4 - 10.8	x10E3/uL	

Annual Labs: Lipid Panel

A Lipid Panel measures fatty substances that your body uses for energy. Typically on a basic Lipid Panel are cholesterol, triglycerides, HDL and LDL.

TEST	LABS	RANGE	UNITS	PERSONAL DATA
LIPIDS	HDL	STANDARD >39 OPTIMAL >50	mg/dL	
	LDL	STANDARD 0- 99.0 OPTIMAL (IT'S COMPLICATED)	mg/dL	
	Triglycerides	STANDARD 0.0 -149.00 OPTIMAL <100	mg/dL	
	VLDL	STANDARD 5.0 - 40.0 OPTIMAL (IT'S COMPLICATED)	mg/dL	

Annual Labs: Urinalysis

Urinalyisis	SPECIFIC GRAVITY 1.005 - 1.030		
	PH 5.0 - 7.5		
	URIINE COLOR	YELLOW	
	APPEARANCE	CLEAR	
	WBC ESTERASE	NEGATIVE	
	PROTEIN	NEGATIVE	
	GLUCOSE	NEGATIVE	
	KETONES	NEGATIVE	
	OCCULT BLOOD	IT DEPENDS	
	BILIRUBIN	NEGATIVE	
	UROBILINOGEN	0.2-1.0 mg/dL	
	NITRITE, URINE	NEGATIVE	

Individual Tests

Individual Tests - these are the specific individual tests we like to review on an annual basis.

Note: µ is the symbol for micro - which can also be abbreviated mc - for example, µg/dL might also be written as mcg/dL - both of which would be said "Micrograms per deciliter."

LABS	RANGE	UNITS	PERSONAL DATA
B-12	STANDARD 232 -1245 OPTIMAL 600- 1200	pg/mL	
C-Peptide	STANDARD 1.0 - 4.4 OPTIMAL 0.5 - 1.6	ng/dL	
Copper Serum	STANDARD 1.60 - 2.30 OPTIMAL 1.60 - 2.30	mg/dL	
DHEA - S FEMALE	STANDARD RANGE 30-39: 45- 270 40-49: 32- 240 50-59: 26-200 >60 13- 90 OPTIMAL RANGE ANY AGE: 65-380	µg/dL	
DHEA - S MALE	STANDARD RANGE 30'S 120-550 40'S 95 -530 50'S 70-310 >60 42-175 OPTIMAL RANGE: ANY AGE 300-600	µg/dL	
ESR (sed rate) FEMALE	STANDARD 0-30.0 OPTIMAL 0 - 18.0	mm/hr	
ESR (sed rate) MALE	STANDARD 0 - 32.0 OPTIMAL 0 - 20	mm/hr	
Ferritin FEMALE	STANDARD 15- 150 OPTIMAL 30 - 70	ng/mL	
Ferritin MALE	STANDARD 30 400 OPTIMAL 30 - 70	ng/mL	
GGT	STANDARD 0.0 - 65.0 OPTIMAL 10.0 - 30.0	IU/L	
hbA1C	STANDARD 4.8 -5.6 OPTIMAL 4.5 - 5.4	%	

Individual Tests (Continued)

LABS	RANGE	UNITS	PERSONAL DATA
Homocysteine	STANDARD 0.0 - 21.3 OPTIMAL 0.0- 7.20	nmol/L	
hsCRP	STANDARD 0-3.0 OPTIMAL 0 - 1.0	mg/L	
Insulin, Serum (Fasting)	STANDARD 2.6 - 24.9 OPTIMAL 2.0 - 5.0	uIU/mL	
Iron, Serum FEMALE	STANDARD 27 - 159 OPTIMAL 85 - 130	µg/dL	
Iron, Serum MALE	STANDARD 38 - 169 OPTIMAL 85 - 130	µg/dL	
Magnesium Serum	STANDARD 1.60 - 2.30 OPTIMAL 1.60 - 2.30	mg/dL	
Phosphorous (Phosphate)	STANDARD 2.50 - 4.50 OPTIMAL 2.50 - 4.50	mg/dL	
TSH	STANDARD 0.45 - 4.5 OPTIMAL 0.5- 2.0	uIU/mL	
Uric Acid FEMALE	STANDARD 1.4-5.8 OPTIMAL 2.5 - 5.50	g/dL	
Uric Acid MALE	STANDARD 3.7-8.6 OPTIMAL 3.5 - 8.5	g/dL	
Vitamin C	STANDARD 2.50 - 4.50 OPTIMAL 2.50 - 4.50	mg/dL	
Vitamin D 25	STANDARD 30.0 - 100. OPTIMAL 50.0 -100.0	ng/dL	
Zinc	STANDARD 2.50 - 4.50 OPTIMAL 2.50 - 4.50	µg/dL	

Thyroid

TEST	SPECIFIC TEST	RANGE	UNITS	PERSONAL
THYROID (FULL LIST)	T4, free	STANDARD .82-1.77 OPTIMAL 1.00 - 1.50	ng/dL	
	T3, free	STANDARD 2.0-4.4 OPTIMAL 3.0 - 3.5	pg/mL	
	Reverse T3	STANDARD 9.2 - 24.1 OPTIMAL 7.0 - 9.0	ng/dL	
	TSH*	STANDARD 0.450-4.50 OPTIMAL 0.5 - 2.0	uIU/mL	
	Thyroid Peroxidase	STANDARD 0.0 - 34.0 OPTIMAL 0.0 - 6.00	IU/mL	
	Thyroglobulin Antibodies	STANDARD 0.0 - 0.90 OPTIMAL 0.0 - 0.90	IU/mL	

*Note: We find, in most cases, people with hypothyroidism who are on medication feel their best with TSH below 1.0, and in some cases, even below the optimal range low threshold. Dialing in your dosage with your doctor should include finding the range you feel is most optimized.

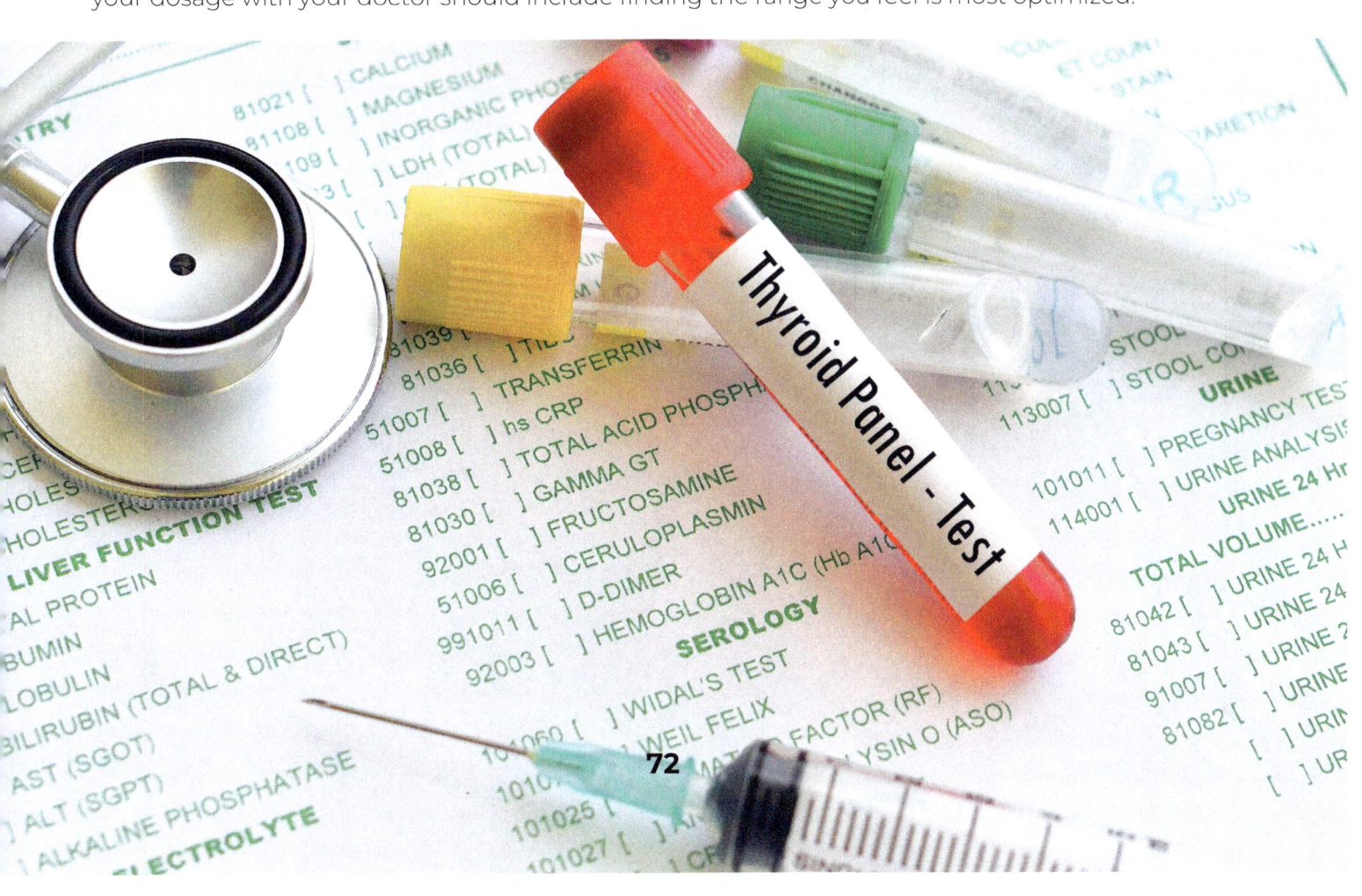

Male Specific Sex Hormones

	LABS	RANGE	UNITS	PERSONAL
	Free Testosterone, direct	STANDARD 9.3-26.5 OPTIMAL SAME	pg/mL	
	Total Testosterone	STANDARD 264.0-916.0 OPTIMAL 500.0-1100.0	ng/dL	
	SHBG (Sex Hormone Binding Globulin)	0-49 Y OLD 16.50-55.9 49+ Y OLD 19.3-76.4 OPTIMAL SAME	nmol/L	
	Zinc*	STANDARD 44.0-115.0 OPTIMAL SAME	µg/dL	
Add if over 50	PSA (Prostate-specific Antigen)	STANDARD 0.0-4.0 OPTIMAL SAME	ng/mL	

*Zinc is not itself a sex hormone, but is implicated in Sex Hormone issues. It is also on the Annual panel, so if adding these to the annual, no need to get it twice!

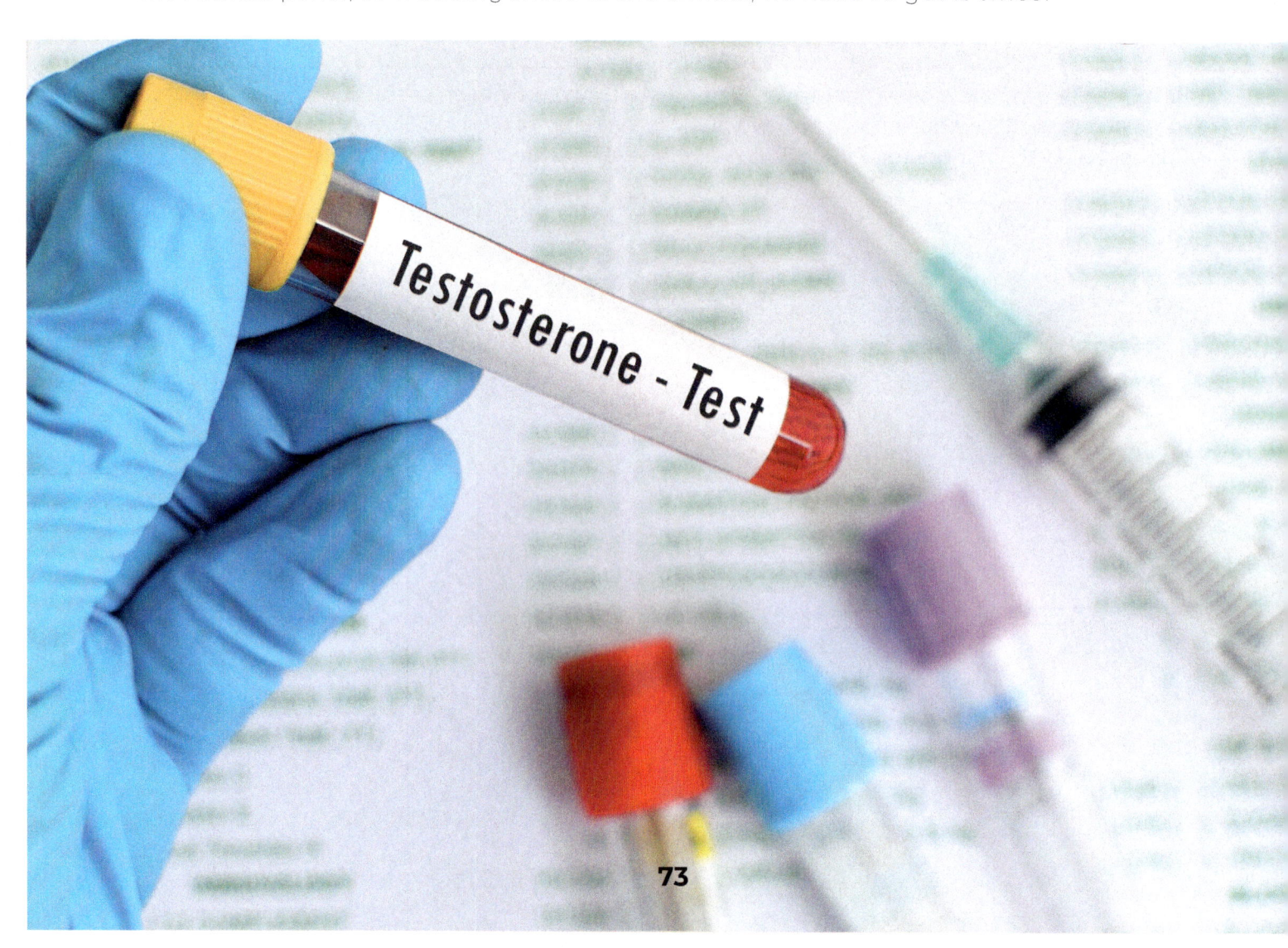

Female Specific Hormones

LABS	RANGE	UINTS	PERSONAL DATA
Total Testosterone	PREMENOPASUAL 10.0-55.0 POSTMENOPASUAL 7.0 -40.0	ng/dL	
Estrodiol	FOLLICULAR PHASE 12.5 - 166.0	pg/mL	
	OVULATORY PHASE 85.8 - 498.0	pg/mL	
	LUTEAL PHASE 43.8 - 211.0	pg/mL	
	POSTMENOPAUSAL <6.0 -54.7	pg/mL	
Progesterone	FOLLICULAR PHASE 0.1 - 0.9	ng/mL	
	OVULATORY PHASE 0.1 - 12.0	ng/mL	
	LUTEAL PHASE 1.8 - 23.9	ng/mL	
	POSTMENOPAUSAL 0.0-0.1	ng/mL	
Sex Hormone Binding Globulin	0-49 Y OLD 24.6 - 122.0 49+ Y OLD 17.3 - 125.0	nmol/L	

Menstrual Cycle Stages	For a 28 day cycle (if longer or shorter, adjust day # slightly)*	Follicular Phase Day 1-7 ish	Day 1= Starts on first day of bleeding
		Ovulatory Phase Day 12-17 ish	
		Luteal Phase Day 18-28 ish	

*A normal cycle can be anywhere from 21 to 35 days, but if you experience changes in average cycle length, make sure to discuss with your doctor!

SECTION 6: COMMON SENSE LAB REFERENCE CHARTS SI UNITS

NOTES ON SI UNITS SECTION

Please be aware that units will vary from country to country on specific tests. This section will list official SI units.

This book was written originally in US units, but we are know many of you are in countries using SI units, so we've added this section with SI units. If your country does not measure in either US/Standard or SI units, there are many online converters that you can use to convert units from this book

Other things to be aware of :

- There can even be differences between labs in the same country, which units were used, and what ranges were consider "normal". So always check the units listed on any test and be certain it's in the same units used on your lab results. If they differ, you can convert them with the aforementioned online calculators.

- Please note that some specific labs are unavailable in some countries. Reverse T3, for example, will not be run in the UK, though some labs there will draw blood for it, then ship the sample to the US for testing.

Annual Labs: CMP

CMP measures blood levels of proteins & electrolytes & glucose levels. These tests reflect the health of your liver, kidneys, bones, muscle cells, nerve and cell funtion.

	LABS	RANGE	UNITS	PERSONAL DATA
CMP	Albumin	STANDARD 35 -55 OPTIMAL 40- 50	g/L	
	Albumin/Globulin Ratio	STANDARD 1.20-2.20 OPTIMAL 1.40-2.10	Ratio	
	Alkaline Phosphotase	STANDARD 39.0 - 117.0 OPTIMAL 70.0 - 100.0	IU/L	
	ALT (SGOT)	STANDARD 0.0 - 44.0 OPTIMAL 10.0 - 26.0	IU/L	
	AST (SGPT)	STANDARD 0.0 - 40.0 OPTIMAL 10.0 - 26.0	IU/L	
	Biliruben Total	STANDARD 0.0 -106 OPTIMAL 8.84 - 79.56	µmol/L	
	Blood Urea Nitrogen (BUN)	STANDARD 2.14 - 8.57 OPTIMAL 4.57 - 7.14	mmol/L	
	BUN/Creatinine	STANDARD 9.0-20.0 OPTIMAL 10.0-16.0	Ratio	
	Calcium	STANDARD 0.48 - 0.57 OPTIMAL 0.51 - 0.56	mmol/L	
	Carbon Dioxide	STANDARD 20.0-29.0 OPTIMAL 25.0-30.0	mmol/L	
	Creatinine	STANDARD 67.19 - 112.27 OPTIMAL 11.97 - 18.81	µmol/L	
	Globulin, total	STANDARD 15-45 OPTIMAL 24 - 28	g/L	
	Glucose (Fasting)	STANDARD 3.6 - 5.5 OPTIMAL 3.6 - 4.78	mmol/L	
	Potassium	STANDARD 3.50-5.20 OPTIMAL 4.00 - 4.50	mmol/L	
	Protein, total	STANDARD 60.0 -85.0 OPTIMAL 69.0 - 74.0	g/L	
	Sodium	STANDARD 134.0-144 .0 OPTIMAL 134.0-144 .0	mmol/L	
	Sodium to Potassium Ratio	STANDARD 30.0-35.0 OPTIMAL 30.0-35.0	Ratio	

Annual Labs: CBC

The CBC looks at levels of components of White and Red Blood cells to evaluate Infections, Allergic Reactions, Blood Volume, Oxygenation, blood clotting and Immune functions.

TEST	LABS	RANGE	UNITS	PERSONAL DATA
COMPLETE BLOOD COUNT (CBC) W DIFF	Baso (Absolute)	STANDARD 0.0 - 0.0002 OPTIMAL SAME	$\times 10^9$/L	
	Basos	NOT ESTABLISHED	%	
	EOS	NOT ESTABLISHED	%	
	EOS (Absolute)	STANDARD 0.0 - 0.0004 OPTIMAL SAME	$\times 10^9$/L	
	Hematocrit	STANDARD 34 -36.6 OPTIMAL 34 - 36.6	%	
	Hemoglobin	STANDARD 111 - 159 OPTIMAL 111 - 159	g/L	
	Immature Grans (Absolute)	STANDARD 0.0 - 0.0001 OPTIMAL SAME	$\times 10^9$/L	
	Immature Granulocytes	NOT ESTABLISHED	%	
	Lymphs	NOT ESTABLISHED	%	
	Lymphs (Absolute)	STANDARD 0.0007 - 0.0031 OPTIMAL SAME	$\times 10^9$/L	
	MCH	STANDARD 26.6 - 33.0 OPTIMAL 26.6 - 33.0	%	
	MCV	STANDARD 79 -97 OPTIMAL 79 - 97	pg	
	Monocytes	NOT ESTABLISHED	%	
	Monocytes (Absolute)	STANDARD 0.0001 - 0.0009 OPTIMAL SAME	$\times 10^9$/L	
	Neutrophils	NOT ESTABLISHED	%	
	Neutrophils (Absolute)	STANDARD 0.0014 - 0.007 OPTIMAL SAME	$\times 10^9$/L	
	Platelets	STANDARD 150-379 OPTIMAL 150 - 379	%	
	RDW	STANDARD 12.3- 15.4 OPTIMAL 12.3 - 15.4	x10E3/uL	
	Red Blood Cells (RBC)	STANDARD 3.77 - 5.28 OPTIMAL 3.77 - 5.28	x10E3/uL	
	White Blood Cells (WBC)	STANDARD 3.4 - 10.8 OPTIMAL 3.4 - 10.8	x10E3/uL	

Lipid Panel

What is often called a Cholesterol test is actually a Lipid Panel. A Lipid Panel measures Lipids in the blood. Lipids are fats and fatty substances that your body uses for energy. Typically on a basic Lipid Panel are cholesterol, triglycerides, HDL and LDL.

TEST	LABS	RANGE	UNITS	PERSONAL DATA
LIPIDS	HDL	STANDARD >1.01 OPTIMAL >1.29	mmol/L	
	LDL	STANDARD 0- 2.56 OPTIMAL (IT'S COMPLICATED)	mmol/L	
	Triglycerides	STANDARD 0.0 -3.85 OPTIMAL <2.59	mmol/L	
	VLDL	STANDARD .056 - 2.22 OPTIMAL (IT'S COMPLICATED)	mmol/L	

Annual Urinalysis

Urinalyisis	SPECIFIC GRAVITY 1.005 - 1.030			
	PH 5.0 - 7.5			
	URIINE COLOR	YELLOW		
	APPEARANCE	CLEAR		
	WBC ESTERASE	NEGATIVE		
	PROTEIN	NEGATIVE		
	GLUCOSE	NEGATIVE		
	KETONES	NEGATIVE		
	OCCULT BLOOD	IT DEPENDS		
	BILIRUBIN	NEGATIVE		
	UROBILINOGEN	0.2-1.0	mg/dL	
	NITRITE, URINE	NEGATIVE		

Individual Tests

LABS	RANGE	UNITS	PERSONAL DATA
B-12	STANDARD 232 -1245 OPTIMAL 600- 1200	pg/mL	
C-Peptide	STANDARD .00331 - .01457 OPTIMAL .00166 - .0053	nmol/L	
Copper	STANDARD 0.056 - 0.128 OPTIMAL SAME	mmol/L	
DHEA - S FEMALE	STANDARD RANGE 30'S 1220 - 7330 40'S 870 - 6540 S50'S 700 - 5430 >60 350 - 2440 OPTIMAL RANGE ANY AGE: 1760 - 10310	nmol/L	
DHEA - S MALE	STANDARD RANGE 30'S 3260 - 14930 40'S 2580 - 14380 50'S 1900 - 8400 >60 1140 - 4750 OPTIMAL RANGE: ANY AGE: 8740 - 16280	nmol/L	
ESR (sed rate) FEMALE	STANDARD 0-30.0 OPTIMAL 0 - 18.0	mm/hr	
ESR (sed rate) MALE	STANDARD 0 - 32.0 OPTIMAL 0 - 20	mm/hr	
Ferritin FEMALE	STANDARD 15- 150 OPTIMAL 30 - 70	ng/mL	
Ferritin MALE	STANDARD 30 400 OPTIMAL 30 - 70	ng/mL	
GGT	STANDARD 0.0 - 65.0 OPTIMAL 10.0 - 30.0	IU/L	
hbA1C	STANDARD 4.8 -5.6 OPTIMAL 4.5 - 5.4	%	

Individual Tests

LABS	RANGE	UNITS	PERSONAL DATA
Homocysteine	STANDARD 0.0 - 21.3 OPTIMAL 0.0 - 7.2	µmol/L	
hsCRP	STANDARD 0 - 3.0 OPTIMAL 0 - 1.0	mg/L	
Insulin, Serum (Fasting)	STANDARD 1.86 X10 - 1.73 X10 OPTIMAL 1.39 X10 - 3.47 X 10	pmol/L	
Iron, Serum FEMALE	STANDARD 4.83 - 28.46 OPTIMAL 15.22 - 23.27	µmol/L	
Iron, Serum MALE	STANDARD 6.80 - 30.25 OPTIMAL 15.22 - 23.27	µmol/L	
Magnesium Serum	STANDARD 0.056 - 0.128 OPTIMAL SAME	mmol/L	
Phosphorous (Phosphate)	STANDARD 0.139 - 0.25 OPTIMAL SAME	mmol/L	
TSH	STANDARD 0.45 - 4.5 OPTIMAL 0.5 - 2.0	uIU/mL	
Uric Acid FEMALE	STANDARD 0.87 - 3.60 OPTIMAL 1.55 - 3.40	mmol/L	
Uric Acid MALE	STANDARD 2.30 - 5.34 OPTIMAL 2.20 - 5.30	mmol/L	
Vitamin C	STANDARD 75 - 250 OPTIMAL 125 - 250	nmol/L	
Vitamin D 25	STANDARD 75 - 250 OPTIMAL 125 - 250	nmol/L	
Zinc	STANDARD 0.139 - 0.25 OPTIMAL SAME	nmol/L	

Thyroid

	LABS	RANGE	UNITS	PERSONAL
THYROID (FULL LIST)	T4, free	STANDARD 10.55 - 22.78 OPTIMAL 12.87 - 19.31	pmol/L	
	T3, free	STANDARD 3.07 - 6.76 OPTIMAL 4.61 - 5.38	pmol/L	
	Reverse T3*	STANDARD 9.2 - 24.1 OPTIMAL 7.0 - 9.0	ng/dL	
	TSH	STANDARD .450-4.50 OPTIMAL 0.5 - 2.0	MIu/mL	
	Thyroid Peroxidase (TPO)	STANDARD 0.0 - 34.0 OPTIMAL 0.0 - 6.00	IU/mL	
	Thyroglobulin Antibodies (TgAb)	STANDARD 0.0 - 0.90 OPTIMAL 0.0 - 0.90	IU/mL	

*Reverse T3 testing is not available in the UK, however some labs will draw blood to be shipped to the US for testing.

Some labs may test in nmol/L - to convert from pmol/L - simply divide by 1000 to convert pmol/L to nmolL

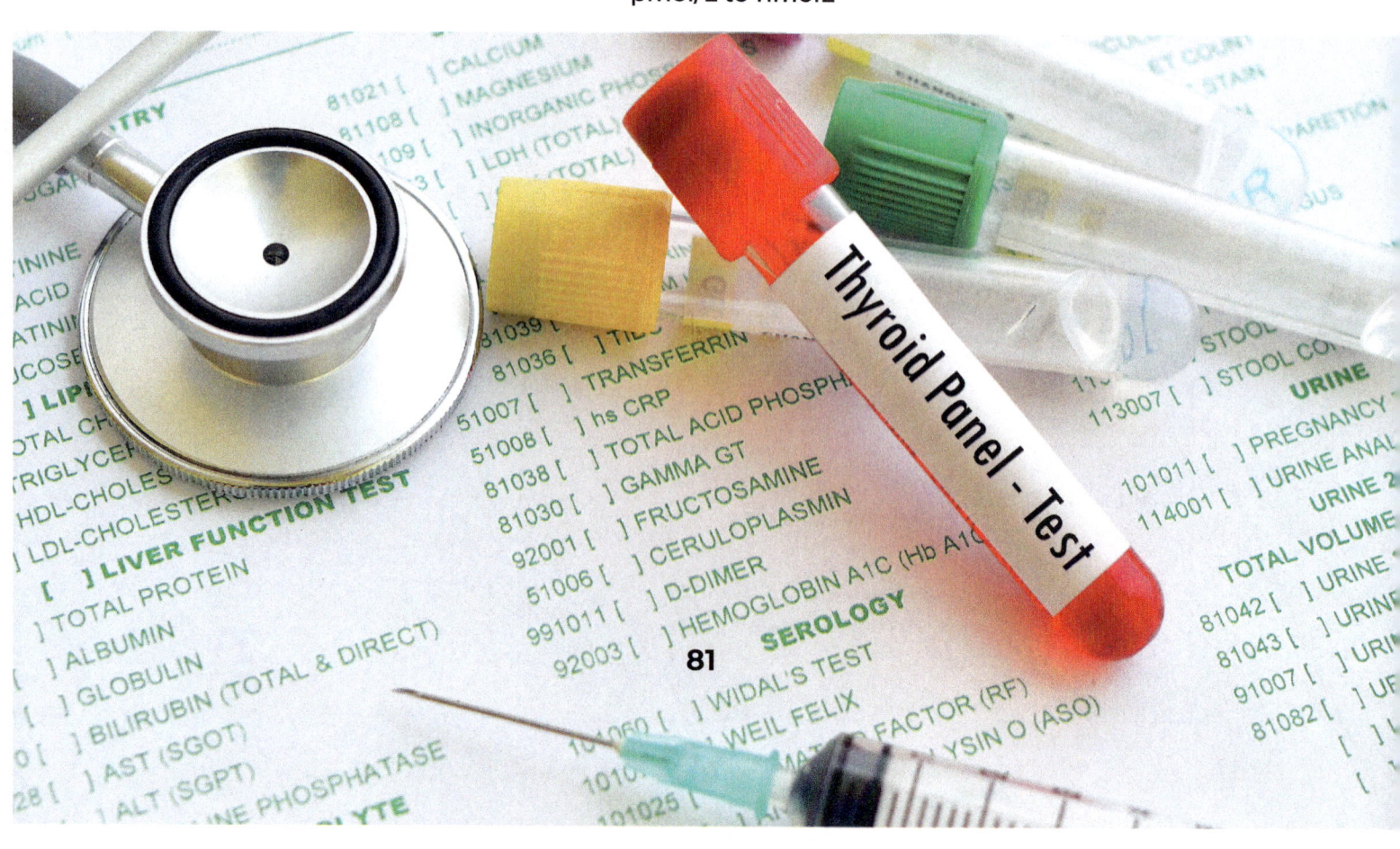

Male Specific Hormones

	LABS	RANGE	UINTS	PERSONAL
	Free Testosterone, direct	STANDARD 32-92 OPTIMAL SAME	pmol/L	
	Total Testosterone	STANDARD 9.2 - 31.8 OPTIMAL 17.3 - 38.1	nmol/L	
	SHBG (Sex Hormone Binding Globulin)	0-49 Y OLD 16.50-55.9 49+ Y OLD 19.3-76.4	nmol/L	
	Zinc	STANDARD 10.02 - 23.99 OPTIMAL SAME	µmol/L	
Add if over 50	PSA (Prostate-specific Antigen)	STANDARD 0.0-4.0 OPTIMAL SAME	ng/mL	

Female Specific Hormones

TEST	LABS	RANGE	UINTS	PERSONAL DATA
	Total Testosterone	PREMENOPAUSAL 0.3 - 1.9 PERIMENOPAUSAL 0.2 - 1.4	nmol/L	
	Estrodiol	FOLLICULAR PHASE 0.128 - 0.373	nmol/L	
		OVULATORY PHASE 0.193 - 0.112	nmol/L	
		LUTEAL PHASE 0.098 - 0.474	nmol/L	
		POSTMENOPAUSAL <0.014 - 0.123	nmol/L	
	Progesterone	FOLLICULAR PHASE 0.00022 - 0.00202	nmol/L	
		OVULATORY PHASE 0.00022 - 0.0270	nmol/L	
		LUTEAL PHASE 0.0041 - 0.0537	nmol/L	
		POSTMENOPAUSAL 0.0-0.00022	nmol/L	
	Sex Hormone Binding Globulin	0-49 Y OLD 24.6 - 122.0 49+ Y OLD 17.3 - 125.0	nmol/L	

Menstrual Cycle Stages	For a 28 day cycle (if longer or shorter, adjust day # slightly)*	Follicular Phase Day 1-7 ish	Day 1= Starts on first day of period
		Ovulatory Phase Day 12-17 ish	
		Luteal Phase Day 18-28 ish	

*A normal cycle can be anywhere from 21 to 35 days, but if you experience changes in average cycle length, make sure to discuss with your doctor!

Thank you!

We see that much of the world goes about life in denial about their declining health. Lack of awareness about what healthy looks like leaves us vulnerable to living a less fulfilling life. People will say, "Oh, that's just part of getting older, can't do anything about it." These beliefs simply normalized poor health.

We've taken it on as our mission to make a stand and tell the world that they do not have to accept others' health limitations as fact. Just because a condition "runs in the family" or "everyone is on blood pressure medication" doesn't mean you have to accept that as your fate. More and more of us are coming to the awareness that rapid health decline doesn't have to be given. When we take steps to change our habits, we change our future.

This book is the culmination of thousands of questions that we have fielded from viewers and subscribers. While it is true that we can't change our genetics or health histories, we can change our expectations of what our best selves can be.
You now have a new set of health tools. You do not have to accept the status quo and can ask more for yourself - and ask for more from your doctor.

This book focused on lab values but we can't stress enough that lab values are not the full picture of health evaluation. How you feel and function is most important, so keep seeking answers if you don't feel quite the way you believe you should. Take the information in this book as a starting point. Use your labs as a snapshot to track your increasing good health over time as you take positive actions towards better health. Track your progress. This is another tool in your toolbox.

Congratulations on taking an active role in better understanding your health. By learning about different aspects of blood lab testing; knowing what questions to ask, and what baseline tests should be checked, you're building a path to a healthier and happier future.
We thank you for taking this journey with us.

In Health,
Dr. Ken Berry & Kim Howerton

Because we know some of you might appreciate studies and articles related to topics in this book as well as links to resources such as blood lab ordering services - we've created a resource page with applicable links for you! It can be found at:

https://commonsenselabslinks.com

ABOUT THE AUTHORS

from Dr. Berry

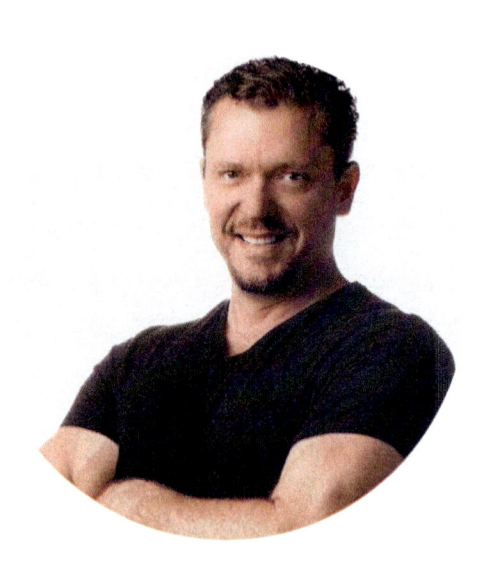

Unlike most doctors, I love questions and ideas from you. I used to be a fat, miserable, ignorant doctor until I slowly discovered the power of removing the slow poisons of the standard diet, and replacing them with the nourishment of a proper human diet...

I am a Licensed Family Physician and have been practicing Family Medicine in rural Tennessee for over 20 years, and have seen over 25,000 patients in my career so far.

No big medical words here, just plain talk you can use to stay healthy and happy. If you like it limp-wristed and sugar-coated then you should probably look somewhere else.

I'll explain how you can use your diet and your lifestyle to get the health you want. Videos about low-carb/ketogenic/carnivore diets, intermittent fasting, thyroid health, hormone optimization, and much more. I've declared an all-out war on the epidemics of hyperinsulinemia, diabetes, and obesity currently hurting our world, and hurting your health.

You can find out more about Dr. Berry at:
drberry.com

from Kim

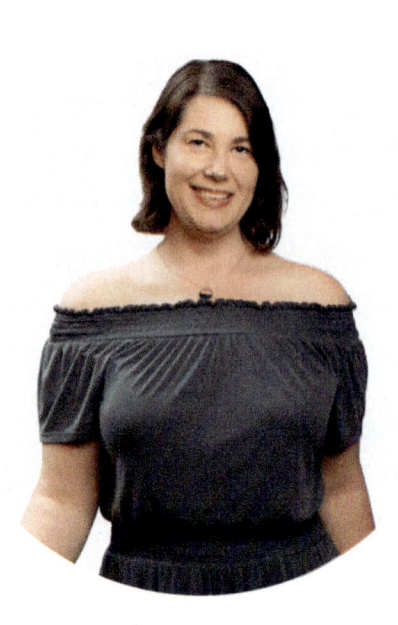

I am a Certified Health & Wellness Coach and recipe creator who works with people who have spent much of their life struggling with their weight and health issues.

On my journey to lose over 100 pounds, I've learned a lot. It was the process of tweaking, unlearning, relearning, experimentation, and deep work that has allowed me to finally feel in control of my health. I credit the messy middle of Keto – where I felt like I was flailing and failing, with the skills that taught me not just to solve my own struggles but to empower others to solve theirs. I now run programs specifically designed for folks who seem to have lost their "easy" button; working with them to find the path to their optimal health.

You can find out more about Kim at:
kimhowerton.com

Printed in Great Britain
by Amazon